KETO AIF

RECIPES

Super Healthy With This Meal Plan for Everyda Cooking

(Easy and Delicious Recipes Perfect for Your Air Fryer)

Geoffrey Givens

Published by Sharon Lohan

Keto Air Fryer Recipes: Super Healthy With This Meal Plan for Everyda Cooking (Easy and Delicious Recipes Perfect for Your Air Fryer)

ISBN 978-1-7776245-9-0

Legal & Disclaimer

The information contained in this book is not designed to replace or take the place of any form of medicine or professional medical advice. The information in this book has been provided for educational and entertainment purposes only.

Table of contents

Part 1

INTRODUCTION

What Is This Book All About?

I will like to welcome you on the voyage that will turn around your whole life for good.

This book consists of established steps and strategies on how to begin preparing healthy and mouth-watering meals that can serve you 24/7 using a single appliance known as the Air Fryer. This improvement creates an opportunity to enjoy fried foods with limited oil. It can equally be used to whip up different categories of dishes, desserts, and snacks.

It contains scores of tasty keto recipes that individuals can tweak in several ways to suit their desire and the types of ingredients obtainable. Each of the recipes has a nutritional value per serving.

Also, it discusses the basics of the appliance, aIR fRYER, and the benefits of using it in contrast to the customary method of frying meal.

Conclusively, the book contains an easy guide of measurement conversion to make your navigation of different types of measurement units across various systems.

Alright, let us begin the journey to healthy living.

CHAPTER ONE

What Is An Air Fryer?

An air fryer uses the convection principle for cooking food. The air fryer passes hot air by using a mechanical fan to cook the foods/meals ingredients inside the fryer. The mechanism bypasses the use of excess oil in the traditional method of frying but still bakes food through a chemical reaction between an amino acid and reducing sugar, often in need of heat; this reaction is known as the Maillard Effect.

The principles were named after a French chemist, Louis-Camille Maillard, who propounded the theory in 1912. The principle gives an uncommon flavor to browned foods like seared steaks, bread, pan-fried meats and fish, biscuits, and cookies, etc.

Amazingly the air fryer only needs a thin layer of oil for food to cook.

The air fryer circulates the hot air within 392^0F.

It is an exceptional way of removing almost 80% of the oil that is traditionally used to fry different meals and make pastries.

There are several arrays of friendly properties in air fryers based on the brand you have. The majority of the brands include temperature control and time adjustment setting to simplify cooking and appliance's ease of utility. It normally has a cooking basket where you position your food. The food basket is set on top of the drip tray.

Depending on the model you have, you will either be instructed to toss the basket to evenly distribute oil or it automatically does that with the help of food agitator without prompting you.

It is excellent for home use, however, if you are preparing a meal for a large number of people and you want to use the same mechanism to cook the food, just place the food ingredients in specialized air crisper tray and bake them utilizing a convection oven. Air fryer and convection oven work on the same principle of cooking but an air fryer has a smaller body and generates low heat.

How To Use Your Air Fryer

There is a manual that comes with the appliance for easy assembly and as a step by step guide for the first users. Lots of the brands also provide you with a booklet of recipes to show you exquisite collections of recipes that you can prepare with your kitchen equipment!

Whenever you want to cook, make sure your food ingredients ready; then place them in the basket and slide it into the fryer. Once the basket is inside, set the temperature and time; the viola begins your cooking!

An air fryer can be used to cook food in several ways, only that you need to master the basics before you try other features, for instance, advanced baking and utilizing air fryer dehydrators. In the same vein, take your time to read and familiarize yourself with all the features contained in the appliance as explained in the manual's guide.

These following under listed are some of the cooking techniques that an Individual can use the appliance for:

1. Fry

It is possible to leave the oil out of your cooking, only that a small quantity will add sweetness and flavor to your meal. You can add oil to the ingredients as you are mixing or spray lightly on the food before cooking. For your health, use the recognized healthy oils such as olive oil, canola oil, avocado oil, peanut, and sunflower oils.

2. Roast

With this appliance, it is possible to get the same quality of roasted foods just exactly as the one cooked in a traditional roaster more quickly. This is suggested for individuals who need to cook a special dish but have a limited time to make a meal.

3.Bake

Certain baking pans are perfectly suited for an air fryer for use in baking cookies, bread, and other pastries.

And this only takes about 15 to 30 minutes to have your baked foods ready.

4. Grill

Air fryer exceptionally grills meals with ease and without difficulties. All you have to do is to shake the basket halfway through the cooking or toss the ingredients once or two times depending on the directives. To make things simple, you can place the ingredients in a grill pan or grill layer with a handle, which comes with the brand or ultimately buy one for your comfort.

There are several types of foods that individuals can cook using an air fryer, only that there also specific types that are not designed for the purpose.

Do not cook ingredients that should and can be steamed for example carrots and beans. Individuals should not fry foods covered in heavy batter in the air fryer.

Apart from those mentioned above, individuals can most types of ingredients using an air fryer. It can be used to cook foods covered in bread crumbs or partially floured. You can similarly cook an array of vegetables in the air fryer, for example, corn on the cob, cauliflower, kale, asparagus, zucchini, and peppers.

It can be used to cook homemade meals and frozen foods by following a variety of instructions outlined for this end.

An air fryer has a separator, a wonderful tool that allows you to cook multiples meals at a time. Make use of separators to divide ingredients in the basket or pan. However, it essential that all of the ingredients have the same temperature setting so that everything will cook uniformly at the same time.

Cleaning The Air Fryer

There is no need to worry about how to clean your air fryer after use, it was primarily designed for trouble-free cleaning.

The components of the fryer are made for non-stick material. This hinders bits of food from attaching to the surfaces which eventually renders it difficult to clean.

It is better to submerge the parts of the equipment before cleaning.

All of the components such as the basket, grill, and pan are designed for easy detachable and cleaning. There is nothing if you soak the parts of the air fryer in dishwater after you have finished cooking your meals.

4 Basic Tips for Cleaning Air Fryer

1. Use specialized detergent for cleaning oil.

2. For perfect and spartan cleaning, let the pan soak in water and detergent for some minutes.

3. Don't use metal utensils to clean air fryer to avoid scratches and scrapes on it.

4. At all times, allow the air fryer to cool off at least 30 minutes before cleaning it.

The Benefits of Air Fryer

It is vital to state categorically that air fried foods remain fried.

only that if you have chosen to get rid of oils in your cooking, you must be watchful about the foods you consumed as this will offer you a better and healthier choice than deep frying. It saves you from unwarranted fats and oils, which eventually helps you to lose weight effortlessly.

1. Cooking with this appliance is not that messy as in the conventional ways of frying. Hence you do not have to worry about greasy spills and stains in your kitchen.

2. It is durable and composed of metal and high-grade plastic.

3. It is built to withstand heavy cooking

4. It can be used to make different meals.

5. It does not give off an unwanted aroma when cooking.

6. It is convenient and simple to use and it is easy to clean.

Cons of Air fryer

Air fryer offers ease and convenience to the kitchen life but there are some headaches attached to them also.

1. Insufficient for large families.

It has a limited basket capability as such cooking meals for a large set of individuals is practically difficult to do at once.

2. The cooking period is longer.

Air fryer cooking took up a larger percentage of time in contrast to traditional deep frying methods. In plain words, air fryer cooking time is two times of deep fryers.

3. It is seriously exorbitant

Because of the perceived value and health benefits connected with the air fryers, some models are so costly than the common deep fryers. For instance, if a deep fryer is sold at $65, there is no doubt air fryer would be sold at $130 or more.

4. It is heavily built.

Air fryers are bulky appliances that occupy large space as such not suitable for small kitchens.

However, efforts are being made to address these limitations in other to make the air fryer one of the most preferred kitchen utensils.

Is Cooking With an Air Fryer Healthy?

Generally, air fryer is construed as a healthy, fun way to relish your cherished 'air' fried meals. They have allegedly reported reducing the fat content of common foods such as chicken wings, French fries, fish sticks, and empanadas, etc.

But just how healthy is cooking with an air fryer?

Air fryers are kitchen utensils that fry foods by the movement of hot air around the foods

Usually, air fried foods are considered healthier than deep-fried foods as they need a small amount of oil to make a related taste, flavor, and texture.

a. Using an Air Fryer Can Help Cut Fat Content

Deep-fried foods are generally higher in fat content than foods produced using other cooking methods.

Air fryers need expressively less fat than conventional deep fryers. Several deep-fried food recipes require about 3 cups of oil, air-fried foods need only just 1 tablespoon.

This indicates that deep fryers use about 50 times more oil than air fryers. Whilst not all of that oil is taken in by the meal, using an air fryer can reduce the total fat content of the food.

Definitely can majorly impact health because higher consumption of fat from vegetable oil has been connected with the risk of conditions such as inflammation and heart disease.

b. Changing to an Air Fryer May Help in Weight Loss

Deep-fried foods are not only higher in fat, but also higher in calories thus a contributory factor to weight gain.

In a study of 33,542 Spanish adults, it was discovered that higher consumption of fried foods was connected with a higher risk of obesity.

Therefore if you are interested in trimming your waistline, switching your deep-fried foods for air –fried foods is the first step in the right direction.

In simple words, air-fried foods are lesser in fat than deep-fried foods, which automatically help lower calorie intake and enhance weight loss.

c. Air fryers can reduce the formation of deadly compounds

Apart from being higher in fat and calories, deep frying dishes can cause possibly harmful compounds such as cyanide, and acrylamide.

Cyanide is produced (in trace quantity) from foods such as lima beans, almonds, pits, and seeds of common fruits such as apples, peaches, and apricots. But frying and smoking may aggravate its effects on the body.

Acrylamide is a chemical substance produced in carbs-rich foods during high heat cooking processes such as frying.

Acrylamide is classified as a "probable carcinogen" according to the International Agency for Research on Cancer. And this implies that certain research indicates that acrylamide may be associated with cancer development.

Though the results are not that validated, some researchers have discovered a link between dietary acrylamide and an increased risk of kidney, endometrial, and ovarian cancers.

Air frying food instead of deep-frying may help decrease the acrylamide content of fried foods.

Although it is essential to be informed that other dangerous substances may still be produced during air-frying. Substances such as aldehydes, heterocyclic amines, and polycyclic aromatic hydrocarbons are all other possibly toxic chemicals that are produced during high-heat cooking and may be connected with a higher risk of cancer. However, further study is still being carried out to determine how air-frying may affect the formation of these substances.

d. Air frying is potentially healthier than deep-frying

In many ways, air-fried foods may be healthier than those deep-fried foods. They are lesser in fat, calories, and even some possibly dangerous compounds that are available in the conventionally fried foods.

If it is your goal to lose weight or reduce your fat consumption without changing or doing away with fried foods, opting for an air fryer may be an excellent decision. However, take note that irrespective of probable health benefits associated with air frying, remember that they are still fried foods.

e. Air-fried food may not be fundamentally healthier

There is no doubt that air-fried foods may be healthier than deep-fried foods, it is necessary to take cognizance of the fact they are closely related to fried food when cooked with oil too. Scores of studies have revealed that consuming fried foods may be connected to several negative effects on health. For instance, a study has established that constantly eating deep-fried foods may be associated with a higher risk of definite types of cancer, including lung, prostate, and oral cancers. Similarly, regular consumption of fried foods has also been linked with type 2 diabetes and hypertension.

So far so good, nothing has indicated that air-frying foods can bring negative effects on the health. It is recommended to cut down on the intake of fried foods to enhance better health.

How Does an Air Fryer Work?

This concept of air frying seems like magic to the uninitiated.

How can one possible fry without fat?

To begin with, air frying is not the same thing as FRYING. Frying implies the submerging of food in oil. There is no other about it. However, an air fryer can provide you with a crispy, crunch that is so mouthwatering.

An air fryer is closely related to a countertop convection oven. It is a small electric utensil with a heating element and fat that circulates air around the cooking chamber. Nevertheless, in the air fryer, the air is undulated very rapidly in a rotational manner. This enables the air to do a better job getting into all the surfaces and crevices of the foods thereby creating a crunchy layer. Also, because the food sits in a holed basket which increases its surface area contact with hot vibratory air. Also, because of the little space that existed the chamber walls, give the basket the capacity to step up the heat.

Frequently Asked Questions (FAQs)

Do you put oil in an air fryer?

Yes of course. But this is the thing, the air fryer can cook food efficiently with just a tablespoon of oil or a spray of oil. And according to the considered views of the nutritionists, air fryer is the best method of cooking that enhances healthy living. If you don't want to use oil, you will be fine. Only that you should see to it that you constantly shake the air fryer to prevent sticking.

What food can you cook with an air fryer?

The type of food you can cook with an air fryer is limitless. Whether it is fresh vegetables or frozen foods, the air fryer is a wonderful cooking appliance that will give you exotic dishes.

Are there any deserts lover?

The air fryer can cook just anything you want to. It is your responsibility to follow your recipes for amazing results. We have included the best air fryer dessert recipes for your sweet tooth.

Is an air fryer worth it?

Definitely yes. It is very fast at cooking and healthier too.

It does not take up much space in your kitchen like your oven, fridge, and stove.

Are air fryers healthy?

As described above it is has been proven beyond a reasonable doubt that air fryer is the healthier alternative method of making dishes.

It lowers cholesterol and calorie intake in contrast to other methods of cooking. There have negative effects of consuming deep-fried foods, ranging from heart problems, thrombosis, obesity, and liver complications.

Is an air fryer the same as a traditional oven?

They are distinct because air fryer can grill, heat leftovers. A traditional oven is larger, hence it can cook enormous cooking.

Is an air fryer better than an oven?

This is difficult to say. But the truth is that both the oven and the air fryer have their own merits and demerits. The air fryer saves time and gives room for different cooking methods to make a variety of delicacies.

However, the oven also cooks food very well and permits cooking in large quantities. It is right to say that they just carry out different cooking roles to the best of their inbuilt ability.

Do you need an air fryer if you have a normal oven?

If you have the means, it is certainly a must-have. This is not to say the oven does not good but the air fryer is not just an appliance for cooking great meals but it also makes kitchen life is so easy, hence you need one.

Is an air fryer the same as an oven?

These two utensils similarly do function but they are different in terms of size and mechanisms.

Do air fryers cause cancer?

The air fryer has not been linked to any effects such as cancers. The air fryer is not known to produce any magnetic rays or chemicals on the food. It only produces heat to the food and heat emission on food has never been connected to any sicknesses not to talk of cancers.

The heat generated by the air fryer is not that high like in other high heat cooking techniques that cause the formation of acrylamide.

Are air fryers toxic?

Not at all if you follow the instructions and guidelines on its usage. Hygiene is very essential for your air fryer and other kitchen utensils.

Is air fried food healthier?

Yes, it is healthy. Several health benefits of this wonderful device have been described in this blueprint.

Does an air fryer make food crispy?

As crispy as you desire! Be it a tender crunch that just melts between your teeth or crunchiest crunch you will have it delivered to you by air fryer.

Is an air fryer good for keto?

Air fryers are good for keto.

Can you use aluminum foil in the power air fryer oven?

Yes! Only that they are instructive tips to follow when using aluminum foil. For instance, you should not place the aluminum foil right at the bottom of the pan because dirt and grease will accumulate there.

Also, make you lay the aluminum foil in a way that does not hang out of the edge of the air fryer basket.

Also, do not lay out the aluminum foil without putting food on it because the aluminum foil gets attach to the heating element and eventually burning.

Can you put a liquid in an air fryer?

Yes, you can but you need to careful with the amount.

Do you have to spray an air fryer?

This is a matter of choice. Spraying distributes oil uniformly and also prevents excess oil in meals.

CHAPTER 2

A Journey Into World of Ketogenic Diet

Beginning a new diet or lifestyle is a procedure that brings a lot of questions irrespective of what diet is or the person involved. There is no doubt making serious changes to one's diet can be so cumbersome and hazy though it should be like this if individuals acting based on the right information. As we all know, if we are armed with correct and update information about any action we intend to take, there is much tendency to be more confident and self-assured.

The first condition to starting the ketogenic diet is understanding what keto stands for. Ketogenic can be described as a process in the body known as ketosis, through which the body burns fat as fuel (energy) in place of sugar. For individuals to attain a state of ketosis, they have to follow solely a low-carb, no-sugar diet that is high in fats and moderate proteins. This ultimately helps the body change its erstwhile process of storing fats and then begin burning them for the energy needs of the body. ketogenic can be a swift and exceptional method of losing weight and promote health.

And because the ketogenic diet is premised on fat burning, it goes to consume extra fat stored in the body and thus helps people get rid of excess baggage of weight and also tone muscle mass.

Similarly, it has been reportedly confirmed keto diet offers hope for individuals who are suffering from seizures, reducing the risk of cardiovascular disease and promote general wellness.

Apart from the burning of stored fats, ketosis impacts a neurological effect that induces happiness and reduced hunger.

What Is A Ketogenic Diet?

A ketogenic diet can be simply defined as a complete plan of eating foods that are high in fat, moderate in protein, and low in carbs.

The ketogenic diet is fundamentally scientific in its performance because it is designed to subject the body to a state of ketosis. Ketosis is a state attained when the body stops burning sugars for energy and begins burning fats as energy.

Fundamentally, a keto diet induces the production of ketone bodies by the liver, hence changing the metabolism of the body from utilizing sugar as the basic source of energy to use of fat as the primary source of energy.

For this process to occur, the keto diet limits carbs consumption below a specific range: generally 100g in a day. Nevertheless, the day to day requirement depends on individuals' health and weight loss goals.

The Mechanism of A Ketogenic Diet

Every single person on the surface of the earth needs food to meet their energy needs. Generally, for a high-carb diet, the body uses sugar as the primary energy source and it is quite easy for the body to change carbs into glucose in contrast with other energy sources.

Also, insulin will be secreted to act on the glucose in the bloodstream and the fats will become store in the body, which ultimately opens the floodgate of several health problems.

However, the ketogenic diet permits the body to utilize another source of energy for fuel.

The whole process is that with lower carb intake, the body will not have adequate glucose it requires and will then be forced to utilize fats in place of glucose, having entered into a condition referred to as ketosis.

Ketosis, a natural state of the body whereby the liver will metabolize the fats obtainable instead of glucose or carbs. Ketones will be produced which will eventually be used by the body as a primary energy source. The major aim of the ketogenic diet is to forcefully subject the body into this metabolic condition.

The human body is naturally designed to adjust to this metabolic state effortlessly. Therefore there is no need to put yourself under mental strain, just allow your body to run its course naturally.

A ketogenic diet is different from other low-carb diets. The difference is that a keto diet primarily consists of 70 to 75 percent of calories from fats, 20 to 25 percent from protein, and 5 to 10 percent from carbs per day.

By abiding with these rules the diet will be made up of high-fats and moderate protein consumption, and as such, there is no need for calorie counting.

As you can see, protein is restricted because it influences insulin and blood sugar in the body. Protein intake in large quantities also leads to excess being converted into glucose. and consequently, the body will get into a state of ketosis.

Naturally, when individuals long for foods, they go for carbohydrates-high foods. This is because the brain has recognized the starchy and sugary foods as "comfort foods".

Hence the principal focus of the ketogenic diet is to greatly reduce the consumption of carbs and adopt a healthier mode of eating. Theoretically, when there is a restriction of carb intake and entering into a state of ketosis, then the excess weight will be eliminated without much ado.

Signs When A body Is In State of Ketosis

There are tests to discover the state of individual ketosis. A body will show visible symptoms when it reached ketosis.

An individual may experience heightened thirst, bad breath (halitosis), loss of appetite, and marked urine smell. All of these are signs given by the body.

1. Digestive problems

Swift change in diet to a ketogenic diet, it is expected to be accompanied by constipation, diarrhea, and other sundry digestive issues.

Though this may vary with individuals and types of foods they choose to eat. It is recommended that individuals should eat fermented foods to improve probiotics and thus enhance digestive health.

2. Increased thirst

The retention of fluid is increased with the intake of carbohydrates. As soon as the carbs are done away with, the water weight is equally gone too. The key is to increase water consumption to prevent dehydration.

Being in a state of ketosis amount to also being in a diuretic state, therefore the need for a large amount of water intake.

3. Reduced Appetite

Definitely reduction of carbs and proteins will lead to increased fat consumption. One is bound to experience a lowered appetite because of the fibrous vegetables, fats, and satisfying nutrients available in the ketogenic diet.

4. The Occurrence of Bad Breath

Individuals may experience metallic taste as well as nail polish odor. This is a byproduct of acetoacetic acid. As the body is becoming more keto-adapted, the bad breath disappears.

5. Keto Flu.

The ketogenic diet can make individuals experience nausea, lethargy, and headache. These effects go away within days. Adding one-half teaspoon of salt into a glass of water will help you taking control of these symptoms.

6. Constipation

During a keto diet, it is essential to drink water sufficiently otherwise one will become constipated due to dehydration.

7. Leg Cramps

Magnesium loss can be difficult to put up with and thus causes pain during the early days of ketogenic diet adaptation.

8. Heart Palpitations

Dehydration may bring about difficulties in breathing. Take measures to improve your salt intake.

But there is no noticeable improvement within a very short period, please consult your physician immediately.

Benefits of The Ketogenic Diet

1. Increased amounts of good cholesterol.

Biologically speaking, High-Density Lipoprotein is classified as good cholesterol. A ketogenic diet has been recognized to increase the levels of High-Density Lipoprotein (HDL) because the body moved the bad cholesterol (Low-Density Lipoprotein-LDL) to the liver where it is reprocessed and eliminated as bio-waste.

2. Epilepsy

the ketogenic diet is the one that entails high fat, low carb and regulated intake of protein, it thus stimulates the body to burn fat as a basic source of energy, This has a positive effect on the incidence of epileptic seizures.

3. It reverses type 2 diabetes.

Consuming lots of carbohydrates lead to their break down as simple glucose. When the glucose enters the bloodstream, it increases the blood sugar levels and induces the production of insulin. This production of insulin informs the cells to absorb the glucose and utilize it or keep it as fat for future usage. Prolonged consumption of low-quality carbohydrates can cause insulin resistance. Thank goodness for the ketogenic diet. The ketogenic diet helps reverse this vicious cycle of the insulin-roller coaster.

5. Quick, lasting weight loss and slimmer waistlines.

The ketogenic diet helps to eliminate all kinds of excess water from the body. Similarly, because it reduces insulin levels, the kidneys begin to remove excess sodium which consequently brings about swift loss of weight with the first two weeks of keto-adaptation.

The ketogenic diet is exceptional at lowering visceral fat as such the waistline quickly shrinks within a very short time of following a ketogenic diet.

6. Improved mental clarity

When a body is in a state of ketosis, there is generally increased inflow of ketone bodies to the brain, thus enhancing brain levels of mental health and focus.

7. Reduced incidence of acne.

A ketogenic diet is known to dramatically lessen the appearance of acne.

8. Improved Strength and Performance

With the ketogenic diet, there is always marked and improved stamina and endurance because of the availability of fat storage as an energy source.

9. For treating Alzheimer disease

The supply of ketone bodies when a body is in ketosis to the brain greatly reduces the overreliance of the brain on glucose, a major source of this disorder.

10. Aging reversal.

The ketogenic diet makes a person looks younger and fresh than his/her age is a catalyst that lessens triglycerides, compound recognized for bringing about scores of the terminal and age-related diseases.

Foods to eat and foods not eat under the Ketogenic diet

Generally, a ketogenic diet encourages a healthy intake of good fats, excellent proteins, and quality carbohydrates. Hence consume fish, beef, pork, poultry, seafood, etc. Be choosy with carbs because of its restriction to little net grams, hence go for leafy veggies and berries due to their low carbs content and high vitamins, minerals, and antioxidants.

The types of food to stay away from in ketogenic diet as clear as day and will be listed here too.

Foods to eat

Vegetables

It is recommended that you opt for green vegetables. Non-starchy vegetables like Brussels sprouts, broccoli, cabbage, cauliflower, lettuce, and zucchini. Avoid starchy veggies such as beans, winter squashes, potatoes, and corn.

Avocadoes

These are a perfect keto staple because they are generally low in carbohydrates, full of nutrients, and rich in healthy fats. They go along with lots of dishes and also an excellent technique to add sweetness and fat to the diet.

Sweeteners

The most common all-natural, low carb sugar replacements are stevia and erythritol. However, experiment to see what suits your system.

Salt.

There is a possibility to experience a reduction in sodium when individuals are following a ketogenic diet.

Himalayan salt, kosher salt, and sea salt are ideal for you.

Nuts.

In moderate amounts, nut and nut butter are an excellent source of fat. Always go for nuts that are high in good fat and low in carbs such as pecans, walnuts, almonds, and macadamia nuts. Be mindful of sunflower seeds, cashews, and pistachios because of their higher carbohydrate content.

Dairy

Cream cheese, grass-fed butter, sour cream, whipping (heavy cream), and cheeses are all good in keto meals. Steer clear of dairy products with added sugars, low fat, and fat-free.

Eggs

We recommend free-range and organic eggs if affordable.

Fats and oils

ghee, butter, beef tallow, olive oil, avocado oil, MCT oil, lard, and coconut oil are healthy fats that should be part of the keto lifestyle.

Meats

Ground beef, chicken thighs, steaks.

Nut flours

Coconut and almond flours tower the chart of keto subs for wheat flour because they are gluten-free, grain-free, and low in carb content.

Fish

Tilapia, salmon, cods, shrimps, and mahi-mahi

CHAPTER 3

BREAKFAST RECIPES

Keto Casserole

Serves-8

Prep Time: 10 minutes

Cook Time: 15 minutes

Total Time: 25 minutes

Ingredients

1lb. ground sausage

½ cup shredded cheese

1 teaspoon fennel seed

½ teaspoon garlic salt

¼ cup chopped white onion

1 diced green bell pepper

8 whole eggs, beaten

Directions

Add the pepper and onion to a skillet; cook in conjunction with the ground sausage until the veggies are soft and the sausage is done.

Spray the air fryer pan with non-stick cooking spray.

Put the ground sausage mixture into the bottom of the pan.

Top uniformly with cheese.

Pour the beaten eggs equally over the cheese and sausage.

Add the garlic salt and the fennel seed uniformly over the eggs.

Add fennel seed and garlic salt evenly over the eggs.

Place the pan directly into the basket of the air fryer and cook for 15 minutes at 390^0F.

Remove the pan gently.

Serve.

Per Serving

 Calories: 282

Total Fat: 23g

Saturated Fat: 8g

Cholesterol: 227mg

Sodium: 682mg

Carbs: 3g

Fiber: 0g

Sugar: 2g

Protein: 15g

Keto Mushroom Breakfast Casserole

Serves- 2

Prep Time: 15 minutes

Cook Time: 20 minutes

Total Time: 35 minutes

Ingredients

½ cup shredded Cheddar cheese

2 tablespoons red bell pepper, chopped

1 green onion, cut

¼ pound breakfast sausage wholly cooked and crumbled

4 eggs, lightly beaten

1 pinch cayenne pepper (optional)

Cooking spray

8 ounces Mushrooms, sliced

Directions

Combine the cheddar cheese, sausage, eggs, onion, cayenne, and bell pepper in a bowl; then toss to mix.

Preheat the air fryer to 360^{0}F.

Spray a nonstick 6-by-2- inch cake pan with cooking spray.

Put the egg mixture in the prepared cake pan.

Cook in the air fryer until set, about 18 to 20 minutes.

Serve.

Per Serving

Calories: 380

Total Fat: 27.4g

Saturated Fat: 12.0g

Cholesterol: 443mg

Sodium: 694mg

Potassium: 328mg

Total Carbs: 2.9g

 Fiber: 0.4g

Protein: 31.2g

Sugars: 1g

Spinach and Egg Spinach Casserole

Serves- 8

 Prep Time: 5 minutes

Cook Time: 12 minutes

Total Time: 17 minutes

Ingredients

6 large eggs

1 teaspoon of olive oil

1 teaspoon of garlic

2 cups of spinach

½ cup of heavy cream

½ cup of cheddar

½ pound of breakfast sausage

Directions

Heat a nonstick skillet to medium-low.

Add the ground breakfast sausage; then bake for about 12 to 16 minutes or until well cooked and browned.

Beat the sausage with a wooden spoon or any utensil of choice.

Remove the breakfast sausage from the skillet and let it cool.

Add 1 teaspoon each of garlic and olive oil to the skillet.

Bake until the garlic is sweet-smelling.

Add the spinach to the skillet and cover; then cook for 5 minutes.

Remove the spinach from the pan and let it cool just like the sausage too.

Add the milk and the eggs together in a medium bowl.

Toss until combined.

Fold in the cheddar, breakfast sausage, and spinach.

Set the silicone muffin cups into the air fryer basket and adjust the temperature to 300^0F.

Fill the cups with the egg mixture, do not fill to the extreme.

You can use a measuring cup to fill the muffin cups.

Set the air fryer time to 12 minutes.

Remove when it is done.

Serve and enjoy!

Per Serving

Calories: 195

Carbs: 7g

Protein: 13g

Fat: 12g

Saturated Fat: 6g

Cholesterol: 191mg

Sodium: 265mg

Potassium: 197mg

Fiber: 1g

Air Fried Breakfast Cups

Serves-8

Prep time: 9 minutes

Cook Time: 15 minutes

Total Time: 30 minutes

Ingredients

¼ cup ground breakfast sausage

¼ cup turnip

¼ cup onion

¼ cup kale

 6 large eggs

2 tablespoons coconut milk

Nonstick cooking spray

Salt and pepper

Directions

Heat a large skillet over medium-high heat

Add the sausage to the pan and bake through, dismantling any big pieces.

When done, remove the skillet and keep aside.

Don't clean the skillet.

Whilst the sausage cooks, peel the turnip and chop into small.

Dice the onion into small pieces.

Remove the stem from the kale; then cut the leaves.

In the same skillet used for the sausage, if it is dry, add 1 tablespoon of olive oil over medium-high heat.

Add the chopped potato to the skillet and bake for minutes or until fork-tender.

Add the onions to the skillet and continue cooking for about 2 minutes, stirring constantly.

Lightly season with pepper and salt.

Remove the skillet from the heat and stir in the kale.

Keep aside.

Whisk together coconut milk, eggs, and nutritional yeast in a large bowl.

Gently fold in cooked sausage, onion, kale, and potatoes until well mixed.

For easy cleaning after use, line the air fryer basket with foil.

Put the silicone baking cups in the fryer basket in one layer. You may work in batches depending upon the size of the air fryer.

Spray cups with non-sticking cooking spray.

Cautiously pour in a ¼ cup of the egg mixture into each cup.

Set the air fryer to 300^0F.

Then fry for 10 to 20 minutes or until the egg is cooked through.

Allow the cups to rest at least 5 minutes before removing them from baking cups.

Serve and Enjoy!

Per Serving

Calories: 380

Total Fat: 27.4g

Saturated Fat: 12.0g

Cholesterol: 443mg

Sodium: 694mg

Potassium: 328mg

Total Carbs: 2.9g

Fiber: 0.4g

Protein: 31.2g

Sugars: 1g

Breakfast Scotch Eggs

Serves- 6

Prep Time: 15 minutes

Cook Time: 15 minutes

Total Time: 30 minutes

Ingredients

Dipping Sauce:

3 tablespoons Greek yogurt

2 tablespoons mango chutney

1 tablespoon mayonnaise

⅛ teaspoon salt

⅛ teaspoon pepper

⅛ teaspoon curry powder

⅛ teaspoon cayenne pepper, optional

Scotch Eggs:

1 pound pork sausage

6 eggs, hard-boiled and shelled

⅓ cup coconut flour

2 eggs, lightly beaten

1 cup panko bread crumbs

Cooking spray

Directions

Add the mango chutney, yogurt, curry powder, mayonnaise, cayenne, salt, and pepper together in a small bowl. Toss to combine very well.

Share the pork sausage into 6 equal portions.

Smooth each portion into a thin patty.

Put one egg in the center and wrap the sausage around the eggs, closing all sides.

Place the eggs aside on a plate.

Preheat air fryer to 390^{0}F.

Add the flour into a little bowl and beaten eggs into a different small bowl.

Put the panko bread crumbs on a plate.

Dip each sausage-wrapped egg into the flour, then dip into beaten egg and allowing the excess skim off.

Roll in bread crumbs and put in a plate.

Spray basket of the air fryer with cooking spray.

Put the eggs into the basket.

Don't overload the basket.

Cook in batches if needed.

Cook for about 12 minutes, turning eggs over when it is halfway to ready.

Repeat the process with the remaining eggs,

Serve with dipping sauce.

 Per Serving

Calories: 407

Total Fat: 27.8g

Saturated Fat: 8.8g

Cholesterol: 284mg

Sodium: 945mg

Potassium: 308mg

Carbs: 21.5g

Fiber: 0.4g

Sugar: 3g

Protein: 21.4g

Breaded Air Fryer Pork Chops

Serves- 2

Total Time-

Ingredients

2 bone-in center-cut pork chops

1 large egg

1/3 cup Panko

1/3 cup seasoned whole wheat bread crumbs

Ghee spray or other high heat cooking spray

Salt and pepper to taste

Butter lettuce, for serving, optional

Directions

Take out the pork chops from the fridge and allow them to stand at room temperature for at least 15 minutes.

In a large deep bowl, whisk the egg.

Combine the whole wheat bread crumbs and panko in another shallow bowl.

Stir to combine very well.

Dip each pork chop in the egg and then press both sides into the bread crumb mixture.

Preheat the air fryer to 400°F.

Grease each pork bite with oil and put in the air fryer in one single layer.

Air fry for 12 minutes, turning over half done until the pork bites become golden brown with an internal temperature of 145°F.

To taste season with pepper and salt.

Serve and enjoy with a side of butter lettuce.

Per Serving

Air Fried Quiche

Serve-

Ingredients

½ refrigerated pie crust

1 large egg

¼ cup milk

½ teaspoon salt

½ teaspoon pepper

1 slice bacon (cooked and diced)

¼ cup shredded Swiss cheese

2 tablespoons minced scallions

Directions

Slice the pie crust to fit into the pan.

Scissors may be used to cut them into correct sizes.

Add the bottom of the dough, put the diced bacon.

Then spread the shredded cheddar cheese and crushed scallions on top of the bacon.

Break 1 egg into a little bowl.

Add the milk.

Add the pepper and salt to taste.

Beat very well.

Pour over the other ingredients; put in the air fryer basket at 320^0F, for 12 minutes.

Allow cooling, then take out of the air fryer basket.

Serve.

Enjoy!

Per Serving

Air fried Omelet

Serve-

Ingredients

2 eggs

¼ cup milk

Pinch of salt

Fresh meat and veggies, chopped- ham, mushrooms, red bell pepper, and green onions

1 teaspoon McCormick good morning breakfast seasoning

¼ cup shredded cheese

Directions

Mix the eggs and the milk until well mixed in a small bowl.

Add a dash of salt to the egg mixture.

Add the veggies to the egg mixture.

Pour the egg mixture into a well-coated 6x3-inch pan.

Put the pan into the basket of the air fryer.

Set the temperature to 350^0F.

Cook for about 8 to 10 minutes.

When you are halfway ready, sprinkle the breakfast seasoning on the eggs and then sprinkle the cheese over the top.

Use a thin spatula to free the omelet from the sides of the pan and move to a serving plate.

Garnish with additional green onions if desired.

Serve.

Per Serving

Air Fryer Quesadilla

Serves-1

Prep Time: 5 minutes

Cook Time: 10 minutes

Total Time- 15 minutes

Ingredients

½ cup shredded cheddar cheese

½ cup shredded chicken

2 (6- inches) flour or tortillas

Cooking spray

¼ cup chopped spinach

Directions

Preheat air fryer to 400°F.

Generously spray one side of one tortilla with cooking spray; then lay flat in the air fryer basket.

Spread half of the cheddar cheese on top of the tortilla.

Top the cheese layer with the spinach and the shredded chicken.

Spread the rest of the cheese over top.

Put the second tortilla on the top of the fillings and spray the top with cooking spray.

Air fry until cheese is melted and tortillas are crunchy about 10 minutes.

Serve.

Per Serving

Calories: 1423

Total Fat: 30g

Saturated Fat: 13g

Cholesterol: 107mg

Sodium: 690mg

Total Carbs: 221.5g

Fiber: 9g

Sugars: 1.1g

Protein: 61g

Air Fryer Egg Rolls

Serves-6

Prep Time: 20 minutes

Cook Time: 18 minutes

Total Time: 53 minutes

Ingredients

2 tablespoons olive oil

1 (1 inch) piece fresh ginger, grated

1 tablespoon minced garlic

10 cooked shrimp, minced

1 egg

12 egg roll wrappers

Cooking spray

1 carrot

¼ cup chicken broth

2 tablespoons reduced-sodium soy sauce

1 tablespoon white sugar

1 cup shredded Napa cabbage or green cabbage

1 tablespoon sesame oil

Directions

Heat the olive oil in a skillet over medium-high heat.

Bake the garlic and ginger until sweet-smelling about 30 seconds.

Add the carrot to the garlic and garlic; bake over high heat for 2 minutes.

Stir in the soy sauce, sugar, and chicken broth into the carrot mixture; then bring to boil.

Add the cabbage; simmer until the cabbage is tender, about 5 minutes.

Take the skillet away from the heat and then stir in the sesame oil

Let the mixture cool for 15 minutes.

Drain the cabbage and the broth mixture.

Fold in the minced shrimp gently.

Break the egg into a small bowl; then whisk.

Fill each egg roll wrapper with the shrimp mixture, putting the shrimp mixture just under the middle of the wrapper.

Fold the bottom point over the filling and tuck beneath.

Fold in both sides and roll up firmly.

Then seal the wrapper with beaten egg.

Repeat the process until all of the egg rolls are done.

Put the egg rolls in one layer into the greased air fryer basket, doing it in batches as necessary.

Spray the egg rolls with oil.

Cook at 390°F for 5 minutes, flip over, and cook for 5 minutes more.

Serve.

Notes

The filling can be prepared in advance and store in the refrigerator.

Per Serving

Calories: 447

Total Fat: 11g

Saturated Fat: 2g

Cholesterol: 336mg

Sodium: 1939mg

Total Carbs: 43.6g

Fiber: 1g

Sugars: 2.5g

Protein: 40g

Breakfast Radish Hash Browns

Serves- 4

Prep Time: 10 minutes

Cook Time: 13 minutes

Total Time: 23 minutes

Ingredients

1 teaspoon garlic powder

1 teaspoon granulated onion powder

¾ teaspoon pink Himalayan salt or sea salt

½ teaspoon paprika

1 pound radishes rinsed

1 medium yellow/brown Onion

¼ teaspoon freshly ground black pepper

1 tablespoon pure virgin coconut oil

Directions

Rinse the radishes very well and chop off the roots.

Trim the stems, allowing ¼ -½ -inch.

Slice the radishes and onion using a food processor or mandolin.

Add the coconut oil and then mix very well.

 Grease the air fryer basket.

Put the onions and the radishes in the air fryer basket.

Cook at 360^0F for 8 minutes, shaking a few times.

Remove the radishes and onions into the mixing bowl.

Add seasonings to radishes and onions.

Cook at 400^{0}F for 5 minutes, stirring halfway through.

Serves.

Per Serving

Calories: 62.81

Fat: 3.68g

Saturated Fat: 3.09g

Sodium: 482mg

Potassium: 313.31mg

Carbs: 7.18g

Fiber: 2.44g

Sugar: 3.32g

Protein: 1.24g

Air Fried Tofu

Serves- 4

Prep Time: 30 minutes

Cook Time: 15 minutes

Total Time: 45 minutes

Ingredients

1 (16-oz) block extra-firm tofu

2 tablespoons soy sauce

1 tablespoon toasted sesame oil

1 tablespoon olive oil

1 clove garlic minced

Directions

Use a tofu press to press tofu at least minutes or placing a heavy skillet on it.

Once done, chop the tofu into small pieces or blocks and add to a bowl.

Combine all of the remaining ingredients into a small bowl.

Sprinkle over tofu; then whisk to coat.

Give the tofu an extra 15 minutes to marinate.

 Preheat the air fryer to 375^0F.

Place the tofu pieces/blocks into the air fryer basket in a single layer.

Then bake for 10 to 15 minutes.

Shaking the pan once in a while to enhance uniform cooking.

Per Serving

Calories: 212

Carbs: 5.2g

Protein: 16.5g

Fat: 15.7g

Saturated Fat: 2.3g

Sodium: 465mg

Potassium: 260mg

Fiber: 2.4g

Sugar: 0.2g

CHAPTER 4

SNACKS AND APPETIZERS

Hasselback Zucchini

Serves-

Ingredients

1 large zucchini, cut in half.

White cheddar cheese

Spices - salt, pepper, garlic, and parsley blend

2 to 10 strips of bacon

1-2 tablespoon of bacon grease

Directions

Preheat the air fryer to 350^0F.

Cut each of the zucchini off.

Stick a chopstick in the center, a little bit off- the middle toward the bottom.

Cut slits into the zucchini.

Season the inside of each slit.

Sprinkle bacon grease on top and a small amount into each slit.

Air fry the zucchini for about 15 to 20 minutes, or until soft.

As the zucchini is cooking, fry about 2 to 4 strips of bacon.

Keep aside to cool.

When the bacon log zucchini is cooked through, remove it, and allow cooling for 2 to 3 minutes.

Begin stuffing the slits with cheese and bacon

When everything is done, add additional cheese and bacon to the top if desired.

Serves.

Per Serving

Calories: 147

Carbs: 6g

Protein: 9g

Fat: 10g

Saturated Fat: 2g

Cholesterol: 49mg

Sodium: 224mg

Potassium: 282mg

Fiber: 2g

Sugar: 3g

Asparagus Fries

Serves- 2

Prep Time: 5 minutes

Cook Time: 8 minutes

Total Time: 13 minutes

Ingredients

16-20 spears asparagus

1/3 cup regular breadcrumbs

¼ cup panko breadcrumbs

1 medium egg

1 teaspoon water

1 tablespoon everything but the bagel seasoning or salt, pepper, poppy seeds, garlic powder, onion powder - 1/8 teaspoon each

Oil spray

Directions

Snap off the hard ends of asparagus, about 1 inch up the stem, and throw away those cut-outs.

Rinse and dry the asparagus using a paper towel.

Add egg and a small amount of water together in a shallow bowl.

Whisk and beat until a bit foamy.

Add the asparagus and toss a little to coat.

In a different bowl, combine panko breadcrumbs, spices, and regular breadcrumbs.

Add the asparagus spears little by little and then whisk until coated.

Place them into the air fryer tray

Repeat until all asparagus are coated.

Place the fries in the air fryer basket; make sure they are overcrowded, work them in batches if necessary.

Spray lightly the tops with oil and then close.

Set an air fryer for 400^0F and 8 minutes.

When it is 5 minutes, open and carefully turn the fries over, then close and bake for the 3 minutes left.

Serve and enjoy with your beloved dipping sauce.

Per Serving

Calories: 127

Total Fat: 4.3g

Saturated Fat: 2.0g

Cholesterol: 39mg

Sodium: 365mg

Potassium: 110mg

Total Carbs: 18g

 Fiber: 2.1g

Protein: 7.5g

Sugars: 3g

Garlic-Roasted Mushrooms

Serves- 4

Prep Time: 10 minutes

Cook Time: 11 minutes

Total Time: 21 minutes

Ingredients

½ teaspoon paprika

1 large egg

12 ounces cremini mushrooms (rinsed and patted dry)

Pure virgin coconut oil (for greasing basket)

Dipping sauce

2 tablespoons butter melted

1 clove fresh garlic minced

2 cups pork rinds

¼ cup parmesan cheese grated

1 tablespoon dried parsley flakes

1 teaspoon garlic powder

¾ teaspoon sea salt

½ teaspoon dried basil

Directions

Rinse the mushrooms judiciously.

Cut off just the bottom of the stem.

Pat dry mushrooms and slice in half.

Break an egg into a medium bowl and toss very well.

Add the mushrooms to the egg wash; then mix to coat entirely.

Add paprika, parsley, pork rinds, parmesan cheese, garlic, basil, and salt to a food processor bowl.

Puree until well combined.

Put the dry mixture in a medium-sized bowl.

Add the mushrooms with the egg wash into the dry mixture; then whisk to coat fully.

Coat the basket of the air fryer with coconut oil.

Add the mushrooms into the basket.

Spray lightly with oil.

Set the air fryer to 380^0F at 10 minutes, turning over the mushrooms when it is halfway ready.

After 10 minutes, increase the temperature to 400^0F.

Then cook for 30 seconds to 1 minute to crunch.

Transfer the mushrooms to a plate.

Serve mushrooms with garlic butter.

Preparing the Dipping sauce:

Mince the garlic and put it into the microwave-safe bowl.

Add butter.

Microwave the butter for 15 to 20 seconds or until melted.

Per Serving

Calories: 132

Fat: 8g

Saturated Fat: 4g

Cholesterol: 71mg

Sodium: 718mg

Potassium: 422mg

Carbs: 5g

Fiber: 0g

Sugar: 1g

Protein: 10g

Baked Zucchini Fries

Serves- 11

Prep Time: 5 minutes

Cook Time: 10 minutes

Total Time: 15 minutes

Ingredients

2 medium zucchini

1 large egg beaten

½ cup or panko/Italian breadcrumbs

½ cup parmesan cheese grated

1 teaspoon Italian seasoning or seasoning of choice

½ teaspoon garlic powder (optional)

Pinch of salt and pepper

Oil for spraying-olive

Directions

Slice the zucchini in half and into fries (also known as sticks) about ½ -inch thick and 3 to 4 inches long.

In a deep bowl, combine the grated parmesan, spices, almond flour (or bread crumbs), and a pinch of salt and pepper.

Mix very well to blend.

Bathe the zucchini in egg and then in the almond flour mixture; then set on a platter or baking sheet.

Liberally spray zucchini with cooking spray.

Working in batches, arrange the zucchini sticks in a single layer in the air fryer.

Cook for 10 minutes at 400^0F or until crunchy.

Serve.

Per Serving

Calories: 147

Carbs: 6g

Protein: 9g

Fat: 10g

Saturated Fat: 2g

Cholesterol: 49mg

Sodium: 224mg

Potassium: 282mg

Fiber: 2g

Sugar: 3g

Air Fryer Biscuits

Serves-9

Prep Time: 5 minutes

Cook Time: 10 minutes

Total Time: 25 minutes

Ingredients

1 cup shredded cheddar cheese

2 large eggs

2 tablespoons butter, melted

1 cup almond flour

½ teaspoon baking powder

¼ teaspoon pink Himalayan salt

2 tablespoons sour cream

Directions

In a large bowl, combine the baking powder, almond flour, and salt.

Add in the cheddar cheese by hand; then mix until well combined.

Add butter, sour cream and eggs to the center; and then blend with a spoon or dirt-free hands until you have a sticky batter.

Place a piece of parchment paper into the air fryer basket.

Put ¼ cup-sized for large or 2 tablespoon-sized for small portions of batter on the parchment paper.

Bake at 400^0F for 6 minutes for small portions to 10 minutes for large portions, until golden brown and cooked through.

Repeat the process for the rest of the batter as necessary.

Serve without delay.

Per Serving

Calories: 167

Fat: 15g

Carbs: 3g

Fiber: 1g

Protein: 7g

Net carbs: 2g

Bacon Jalapeno Popper

Serve- 8

Total Time:

Ingredients

½ cup shredded cheddar

½ teaspoon garlic powder

¼ teaspoon onion powder

4 jalapenos

3 ounces cream cheese, softened

4 slices bacon

Directions

Set the air fryer to 390^{0}F and heat for 2 minutes.

Sensibly add the jalapenos to the air fryer basket in one layer with space between them.

Work in batches if the air fryer cannot contain 8 halves at a go.

Air fry for 10 minutes or until bacon is crispy.

Serve.

Notes

When you are handling jalapenos, it is recommended that you wear gloves so that oil from the peppers does not burn the skin. However, if there are no gloves, rinse your hands very well right after handling peppers.

Per Serving

 Calories: 96

Total Fat: 8g

Saturated Fat: 4g

Cholesterol: 23mg

Sodium: 177mg

Carbs: 1g

Net Carbs: 1g

Fiber: 0g

Sugar: 1g

Protein: 4g

Air fried Keto Hamburgers

 Serves- 2

Prep Time: 5 minutes

Cook Time: 10 minutes

Total Time: 15 minutes

Ingredients

¼ teaspoon onion powder

¼ teaspoon garlic powder

¼ teaspoon smoky paprika

2 strips thin cut bacon

2 (4-ounce) hamburger patties, flattened to ½ inch thickness

½ teaspoon fine grain sea salt

¼ teaspoon fresh ground pepper

Optional Toppings:

2 (1-ounce) slice sharp cheddar cheese (ignore for dairy-free)

2 large butter lettuce leaves

Condiments: Ranch Dressing, mustard, keto ketchup, or mayonnaise

2 slices tomato

1 slice red onion

¼ avocado, sliced

Directions

Preheat the air fryer to 360^{0}F.

Put the bacon into the air fryer.

Cook for 4 to 6 minutes, subject to the thickness of bacon and the level of crispness you desire for the bacon.

In the meantime, combine the garlic powder, onion powder, pepper, and salt in a small bowl.

Stir to blend very well.

Take out the bacon and place aside on a paper towel-lined plate or tray.

Season the patty very well with seasoning mixture.

Put the patties in the air fryer.

Bake for 7 minutes for an averagely-done burger or bake longer if you like a well-cooked burger.

Put the cheese slices on the burgers.

Bake for 1 minute to melt the cheese.

Remove the burgers from the air fryer with a spatula or a ladle.

Serve with lettuce leaves, onion, avocado, bacon, tomato, and condiments of your preference.

It is best served and consumed fresh.

Notes

Extras can be stored in an airtight container in the fridge for 3 days or in the freezers for about 1 month.

To reheat place into air fryer at 350^{0}F for 4 minutes or until heated through.

Per Serving

Calories: 80

Protein: 5g

Carbs: 0g

Fiber: 0g

Sugar: 0g

Fat: 7g

Saturated Fat: 3g

Sodium: 45mg

Old Bay Chicken Wings

Serves- 4

Prep Time: 15 minutes

Cook Time: 25 minutes

Total Time: 40 minutes

Ingredients

2 pounds of chicken wings

2 tablespoons seafood seasoning

¼ teaspoon freshly cracked black pepper

½ cup cornstarch

Sauce:

4 tablespoons butter

1 teaspoon seafood seasoning

Directions

Preheat the air fryer to 400^0F.

Put the chicken wings in a large bowl; add 2 tablespoons seafood seasoning and black pepper to it, and then whisk to coat.

Add the cornstarch and toss the chicken wings until completely coated.

Put each chicken wing in the air fryer basket, ensure that they are not overlapping.

Cook in batches if there is a need.

Cook in the preheated (400^0F) air fryer for 10 minutes, toss the basket and cook for an extra 8 minutes.

Turn the wings over and cook until the chicken is cooked enough and juices run clear, about 5 to 6 more minutes.

In the meantime, in a small bowl, mix butter and 1 teaspoon seafood seasoning for the sauce.

Bring to boil over medium-high heat, stirring frequently.

Dip each chicken wing in the sauce.

Serve with remaining sauce on the side.

Enjoy!

Calories: 335

Total Fat: 22.8g

Saturated Fat: 10.4g

Cholesterol: 78mg

Sodium: 1083mg

Potassium: 139mg

Carbs: 15.8g

Fiber: 1g

Sugar: 0g

Protein: 15.7g

Air Fryer Cauliflower

Serves- 2

Prep Time: 5 minutes

Cook Time: 15 minutes

Total Time: 20 minutes

Ingredients

½ head cauliflower

1 to 2 tablespoons olive oil 15 to 30 mL

Pinch of salt and pepper

Directions

Slice the cauliflower into florets.

Shake with olive oil pepper and salt.

Place in a single layer in the air fryer basket or tray.

Cook at 375°F for 10 to 15 minutes, or until fork-soft and slightly browned.

Serve and enjoy warm.

Per Serving

Calories: 77

Carbs: 3.5g

Protein: 1.3g

Fat: 7.1g

Saturated Fat: 1g

Sodium: 97mg

Potassium: 201mg

Fiber: 1.7g

Sugar: 1.6g

Crispy Keto Pork Bites

Serves- 6

Prep Time: 5 minutes

Cook Time: 12 minutes

Total Time: 17 minutes

Ingredients

¼ cup grated Parmesan cheese

1 teaspoon garlic powder

1 teaspoon Creole seasoning

1½ lb. boneless pork chops

1/3 cup almond flour

1 teaspoon Paprika

Directions

Preheat the air fryer to 360^{0}F.

In the meantime, combine all of the ingredients apart from pork chops into a big Ziploc bag.

Put the pork chops into the bag, close it and then toss to coat the pork chops very well.

Remove from the bag and put it in the air fryer in one layer.

Bake for about 8 to 12 minutes, based on the thickness of the pork chops.

Serve.

Per Serving

Calories: 231

 Carbs: 2g

Protein: 27g

 Fat: 12g

 Saturated Fat: 3g

Cholesterol: 79mg

 Sodium: 118mg

 Potassium: 437mg

 Fiber: 1g

CHAPTER 5

CHICKEN RECIPES

French Garlic Chicken

Serves- 4

Ingredients

¼ cup lemon juice

2 tablespoons olive oil

1 teaspoon Dijon mustard

2 cloves garlic, minced

¼ teaspoon salt

⅛ teaspoon ground black pepper

4 skin-on, bone-in chicken thighs

4 lemon wedges

Directions

Toss the Dijon mustard, pepper, salt, garlic, lemon juice, and olive oil together in a bowl.

Keep the marinade aside.

Put the chicken thighs into a big re-sealable plastic bag.

Pour the marinade on top of the chicken and seal the bag.

Just make sure all parts of the chicken are covered with the marinade.

Chill for at least 2 hours.

Preheat an air fryer to 360^0F.

Take the chicken from the marinade.

Use paper towels to pat dry.

Put the chicken pieces in the air fryer basket.

Cooking may be done in batches if needed.

Cook until the chicken is no longer pink and the juices run clear about 22 to 25 minutes.

An instant-read thermometer inserted near the bone should read 165^0F.

Squeeze a lemon wedge on top of each piece when serving.

Per Serving

Calories: 258

Total Fat: 18.6g

Saturated Fat: 4.2g

Cholesterol: 71mg

Sodium: 242mg

Potassium: 215mg

Carbohydrates: 3.6g

Fiber: 0.7g

Sugar: 0g

Protein: 19.4g

Air Fried Whole Chicken

Serves- 6

Prep Time: 5 minutes

Cook Time: 1 hour

Total Time: 1 hour 5 minutes

Ingredients

1 5 pounds whole chicken, giblets removed

2 tablespoons avocado oil

1 tablespoon kosher salt

1 teaspoon freshly ground black pepper

1 teaspoon garlic powder

1 teaspoon paprika (smoked)

½ teaspoon dried basil

½ teaspoon dried oregano

½ teaspoon dried thyme

Directions

Combine all of the seasoning ingredients with the avocado oil to form a paste.

Spread all the paste over the chicken.

Spray the air fryer basket with cooking spray.

Put the chicken in the air fryer basket breast side down.

Cook at 360^0F for 50 minutes.

Turn over the chicken with breast side up; then cook for extra 10 minutes.

Check to see that the breast meat has an internal temperature of 165^0F.

Serve.

Per Serving

Calories: 478

Carbs: 10g

Protein: 37g

Fat: 33g

Saturated Fat: 12g

Cholesterol: 120mg

Sodium: 780mg

Potassium: 403mg

Fiber: 4g

Sugar: 2g

Southern Fried Chicken Tenders

Serves- 6

Prep Time: 10 minutes

Cook Time: 20 minutes

Total Time: 30 minutes

Ingredients

2½ lbs. chicken drumsticks

1 teaspoon smoked paprika

½ teaspoon garlic powder

¼ teaspoon dried thyme

¼ cup coconut flour

½ teaspoon of sea salt

¼ teaspoon black pepper

2 large eggs

1 cup pork rinds

Directions

In a medium shallow bowl, stir in the coconut flour, black pepper, and sea salt together.

Keep aside.

In another medium-sized bowl, toss together the eggs.

Set aside.

Take a third bowl, combine the smoked paprika, garlic powder, crushed pork rinds, and thyme; mix to blend very well.

Bathe the chicken pieces in the coconut flour mixture, dip in the eggs, dust off the excess, and then press into the pork rind mixture.

For perfect results, keep the majority of the third mixture in a separate bowl, and add a small amount at a time to another bowl dedicated to coating the chicken.

Preheat the air fryer at 400^0F for 5 minutes.

Lightly smear the metal basket and lay the breaded chicken on it in a single layer without overlapping each other.

Set the basket into the air fryer.

Cook for 20 minutes or until the internal temperature is 165^0F.

Serve.

Per Serving

Calories:273

Fat:15g

Protein:28g

Total Carbs:3g

Net Carbs:2g

Fiber:1g

Sugar: 0g

Chicken Piccata

Serves- 4

Prep Time: 5 minutes

Cook Time: 15 minutes

Total Time: 30 minutes

Ingredients

2 (16 oz.) total skinless chicken breasts, all fat trimmed

Freshly ground black pepper, dash

½ cup reduced-sodium chicken broth

1 tablespoon capers

Sliced lemon, for serving

2 large egg whites

2/3 cup seasoned whole wheat dry bread crumbs

Olive oil spray, about 1 tablespoon

1 tablespoon whipped butter

Juice of 1 lemon, lemon halves reserved

¼ cup dry white wine

Chopped fresh parsley leaves, for serving

Directions

Dice the chicken into 4 cutlets.

Put the cutlets between 2 sheets of parchment paper or plastic wrap and pound out to ¼ -inch thick.

Dust both sides with salt and pepper.

In a shallow bowl, beat the egg whites and 1 teaspoon of water together.

Add the bread crumbs to another plate.

Immerse each chicken breast in the egg, then in the bread crumbs.

Place the chicken breasts in the air fryer basket and then generously spray with olive spray. There should be free from one another.

Preheat the air fryer to 370^0F.

Cook for 5 to 6 minutes.

Flipping halfway until crisp and golden and cooked through.

Serve.

Per Serving

Calories: 262

Carbs: 11.5g

Protein: 30g

Fat: 9.5g

Saturated Fat: 2.5g

Cholesterol: 88mg

Sodium: 233.5mg

Fiber: 1.5g

Sugar: 0.5g

Air Fried Chicken Drumsticks

Serves- 2

Prep Time: 5 minutes

Cook Time: 25 minutes

Total Time: 30 minutes

Ingredients

1.5 lbs. chicken drumsticks

1/3 cup almond flour

1 teaspoon of sea salt

½ teaspoon fresh cracked pepper

2 tablespoons olive oil

¼ cup ultra-fine grated parmesan cheese*

Directions

Cream the chicken legs with olive oil.

Then sprinkle with salt and pepper.

Mix almond flour and parmesan.

Spray or oil the air fryer basket with nonstick.

Coat the chicken legs with cheese/flour mixture then transfer to the air fryer basket.

Preheat the air fryer at 400ºF for 25 minutes.

Turn over the chicken legs halfway through the cooking time.

Serve.

Notes

For a super fine powdered parmesan cheese, then pulse the shredded parmesan cheese in a blender.

Per Serving

Calories: 911

Total Fat: 57g

Saturated Fat: 12g

Cholesterol: 443mg

Sodium: 1617mg

Carbs: 6g

Fiber: 2g

Sugar: 1g

Protein: 89g

Crack Chicken

Serves- 4

Prep Time: 5 minutes

Cook Time: 20 minutes

Total Time: 25 minutes

Ingredients

8 chicken skins

½ teaspoon kosher salt

Directions

Use a paper towel to pat dry the chicken skins.

Sprinkle kosher salt on both sides of the chicken skins.

Place the 3 or chicken skin in one single layer with the skin- side down on the air fryer basket.

Set the air fryer to bake at 400°F for 12 minutes.

Flip the chicken skins halfway through, so that they are skin side-up.

Air fryer the chicken skins the remaining 6 minutes or until crispy.

Add 1 or 2 minutes to the cooking period if the skin is somewhat flaccid in parts.

Remove the chicken crack from the air fryer.

Place on a wire rack to cool.

Discard any chicken fat on the bottom of their air fryer before repeating the processes with the remaining chicken skins.

Serve.

Per Serving

Calories: 371

Carbs: 1g

 Protein: 28g

Fat: 28g

Keto Adobo Air Fried Chicken Thighs

Serves- 4

Prep Time: 5 minutes

Cook Time: 20 minutes

Total Time: 25 minutes

Ingredients

4 large chicken thighs

1 tablespoon olive oil

2 tablespoons adobo seasoning

Directions

Add olive oil to a bag or plat and then coat the chicken thighs in it.

Whisk chicken thighs in adobo seasoning to coat.

Put the chicken thighs in the air fryer basket.

Don't let them touch one another.

Set an air fryer to 350^0F and set the timer to 10 minutes.

After 10 minutes, turn over chicken to another side; and then cook another 10 minutes.

Chicken should be golden brown and 165^0F internal temperature when it is cooked through.

Per Serving

Calories: 359

Total Fat: 24g

Saturated Fat: 7g

Cholesterol: 186mg

Sodium: 2616mg

Carbs: 1g

Fiber: 1g

Sugar: 0g

Protein: 36g

Air Fried Lemon Chicken

Serves- 6

Prep Time: 5 minutes

Cook Time: 20 minutes

Total Time: 25 minutes

Ingredients

1 tablespoon Italian herb seasoning blend

1 teaspoon Celtic sea salt

1 teaspoon fresh cracked pepper

6 chicken thighs

2 tablespoons olive oil

2 tablespoons lemon juice

1 lemon, sliced thin

Directions

Put all of the ingredients apart from sliced lemon to bowl; then to coat the chicken.

Allow to marinate for 30 minutes or overnight.

Remove the chicken.

Let any excess oil fall off.

Lay the chicken thighs and lemon slices in the air fryer basket, whilst ensuring that the chicken thighs are free from one another.

Set an air fryer to 350^0F and cook for 10 minutes.

Remove the fryer basket and turn over the chicken thighs to another side.

Cook again at 350^0F for another 10 minutes.

The chicken thighs should be crispy with juices running clear.

Also, the internal temperature should be 165^0F when checked with a digital thermometer inserted in the thickest portion of the chicken thigh.

Serve and enjoy!

Per Serving

Calories: 325

Total Fat: 23g

Saturated Fat: 6g

Cholesterol: 166mg

Sodium: 679mg

Carbs: 2g

Fiber: 1g

Sugar: 0g

Protein: 31g

Air Fried Chicken Tenderloin

Serves: 4

Total Time:

Ingredients

1 pound chicken tenders

1 teaspoon garlic powder

1 teaspoon paprika

½ cup almond flour or coconut flour

1 egg beaten

Salt and pepper to taste

Directions

Spray the air fryer basket with cooking spray very well.

Chicken tenders may stick as such breading will pull for if the air fryer is not sprayed sufficiently.

Add salt and pepper to chicken tenders to season.

Dip the chicken tenders into flour, then egg and then into the flour again.

Set the chicken into the air fryer basket.

Cook at 350^0F for about 5 minutes.

Turn the chicken tenders over; then cook for an extra 5 minutes.

Cook until the internal temperature reads 165^0F.

Serve.

Per Serving

Calories: 299

Carbs: 7g

Protein: 25g

Fat: 19g

Saturated Fat: 2g

Cholesterol: 125mg

Sodium: 815mg

Potassium: 251mg

Fiber: 3g

Sugar: 1g

CHAPTER 6

BEEF

Italian Beef Roast

Serves-

Prep Time: 5 minutes

Cook Time: 1 hour

Total Time: 1 hour 15 minutes

Ingredients

2-pound beef roast

2 teaspoons garlic powder

2 teaspoons onion salt

2 teaspoons parsley

2 teaspoons thyme

2 teaspoons basil

½ tablespoon salt

1 teaspoon pepper

1 tablespoon olive oil

Directions

Preheat the air fryer for 15 minutes at 390^0F.

Combine the parsley, basil, onion salt, garlic powder, and thyme in a bowl.

Rub the herb mixture over the whole roast.

Place the roast in the preheated air fryer.

Set timer for 15 minutes.

After 15 minutes, remove the basket and flip the roast over.

Bring the temperature to down 3600F on the air fryer and return the roast.

Cook another 60 minutes or until the thermometer attains the preferred degree of doneness.

Let roast rest for 15 minutes before slicing.

Serve.

Per Serving

 Calories: 336

Total Fat: 16g

Saturated Fat: 5.5g

Cholesterol: 136mg

Carbs: 1g

Sugar:0g

Protein: 69g

Air Fryer Roast Beef

Serves- 4

Prep Time: 5 minutes

Cook Time: 45 minutes

Total Time: 50 minutes

Ingredients

1 kg beef joint

1 tablespoon extra-virgin olive oil

Salt and pepper

Directions

Remove the roast beef out of the packaging.

Rub the roast beef with extra virgin olive oil.

Then season with pepper and salt.

Put the seasoned roast beef into the air fryer oven rotisserie and attach it in place.

Set the air fryer temperature to 380^0F and time at 45 minutes.

Check to confirm if the beef rotating.

When it is 45 minutes, test to see if it cooked through.

Then slice.

Serve.

Per Serving

Calories: 666

Protein: 43g

Fat: 54g

Saturated Fat: 20g

Cholesterol: 178mg

Sodium: 168mg

Potassium: 675mg

Air Fryer Mongolian Beef

Serves- 4

Prep Time: 20 minutes

Cook Time: 20 minutes

Total Time: 40 minutes

Ingredients

1 lb. flank steak

¼ cup of corn starch

Sauce

2 teaspoons olive oil

½ teaspoon ginger

1 tablespoon minced garlic

½ cup soy sauce or gluten-free soy sauce

½ cup of water

¾ cup brown sugar, packed Adds on

Cooked rice

Green beans

Green onions

Directions

Slice the steak in finely long pieces.

Then coat them with the corn starch.

Put in the air fryer.

Cook at 390^{0}F for 5 minutes per each side.

Whilst the steak cooks, warm up all sauce ingredients in a medium saucepan on medium-high heat.

Toss the ingredients together until it gets to a low boil.

When the steak and sauce are cooked through, put the steak in the same bowl with the sauce; allow it to soak for about 5 to 10 minutes.

Remove the steak with tongs when ready to serve as this will allow the excess sauce to fall off.

Serve.

You may enjoy it with cooked rice and green beans if you desire.

Per Serving

Air Fryer Korean BBQ Beef

Serves- 6

Prep Time: 15 minutes

Cook Time: 30 minutes

Total Time: 45 minutes

Ingredients

1 pound flank steak or thinly sliced steak

¼ cup of corn starch

Coconut oil spray

Sauce

2 tablespoon white wine vinegar

1 clove garlic, minced

1 tablespoon hot chili sauce

1 teaspoon ground ginger

½ teaspoon sesame seeds

½ cup soy sauce or gluten-free soy sauce

½ cup brown sugar

1 tablespoon cornstarch

1 tablespoon water

Directions

Slice the steak finely.

Then toss in the cornstarch.

Spray or line the air fryer basket with coconut oil spray or foil.

Put the steak into the air fryer basket; then spray again to coat.

Bake at 390^{0}F for 10 minutes.

Flip over the steak and then cook for an extra 10 minutes.

Whilst the steak is cooking, add the sauce ingredients apart from the cornstarch and water to a medium-sized saucepan.

Heat it to a low boil.

Then whisk in the cornstarch and water.

Carefully take out the steak and then pour the sauce over the steak.

Mix very well.

Serve.

Garnish with sliced green onions, green beans, and cooked rice.

Per Serving

Calories: 487

Total Fat: 22g

Saturated Fat: 10g

Cholesterol: 113mg

Sodium: 1531mg

Carbs: 32g

Fiber: 2g

Sugar: 21g

Protein: 39g

Air Fryer Steak Bites and Mushrooms

Serves- 4

Prep Time: 10 minutes

Cook Time: 20 minutes

Total Time: 30 minutes

Ingredients

1 lb. steaks, cut into 1-inch cubes and patted dry

Salt, to taste

Black pepper, to taste

Crushed parsley, garnish

8 oz. mushrooms, cleaned, rinsed and halved

2 tablespoons butter, melted or oil

1 teaspoon Worcestershire sauce

½ teaspoon garlic powder

Melted butter, optional

Chili Flakes, optional

Directions

Add the mushrooms and the steak cubes together in a bowl.

Coat with the melted butter.

Season with garlic powder, pepper, Worcestershire sauce, and salt.

Preheat the air fryer at 400°F for 4 minutes.

Place the steak and mushrooms in a single layer in the air fryer basket.

Cook for 10 to 18 minutes, shaking and flipping whilst cooking.

Double-check to see if the steak is cooked through.

If there is a need for more time, an additional 2 to 5 minutes cooking time is proper.

Garnish with parsley and shower with optional melted butter and/or optional chili flakes. Season with extra salt and pepper if desired.

Serve warm.

Per Serving

Air Fryer Cheesy Beef Enchiladas

Serves- 8

Prep Time: 20 minutes

Cook Time: 10 minutes

Total Time: 30 minutes

Ingredients

1 can mild chopped green chilies, drained

1 can red enchilada sauce

1cup shredded Mexican cheese

1 cup chopped fresh cilantro

½ cup sour cream

1 pound ground beef

1 package taco seasoning or gluten-free taco seasoning

8 gluten-free tortillas

1 can black beans, drained and rinsed

1 can diced tomatoes, drained

Directions

Brown the ground beef in a medium skillet over medium heat.

Add the taco seasoning according to the package instructions.

Form each tortilla by beef, tomatoes, beans, and chilies.

Line the air fryer basket with foil.

Put each one inside the air fryer basket

When all the enchiladas are made, pour the enchilada sauce evenly over them.

Equally, add the cheese on top.

Bake at 355^{0}F for 5 minutes in the air fryer.

Remove with care.

Add toppings; then serve.

Per Serving

 Calories: 454

Total Fat: 20g

Saturated Fat: 8g

Cholesterol: 72mg

Sodium: 655mg

Carbs: 40g

Fiber: 6g

Sugar: 2g

Protein: 27g

Air Fryer Steak Fajitas with Onions and Peppers

Serves- 6

Prep Time: 10 minutes

Cook Time: 15 minutes

 Total Time: 25 minutes

Ingredients

1 lb. thin-cut steak

1 green bell pepper sliced

1 yellow bell pepper sliced

1 red bell pepper sliced

½ cup white onions sliced

1 packet gluten-free fajita seasoning

Olive oil spray

Gluten-free corn tortillas or flour tortillas

Directions

To begin with, line the basket of the air fryer with foil and coat with spray.

Finely slice the steak against the grain, about ¼ -inch per slice.

Blend the steak with onions and peppers.

Add to the air fryer.

Evenly coat with the fajita seasoning.

Cook for 5 minutes on 390^0F.

Mix up the steak mixture.

Carry on cooking for an extra 5 to 10 minutes until the desired doneness is achieved.

Serve in warm tortillas.

Per Serving

Calories: 305

Total Fat: 17g

Saturated Fat: 6g

Cholesterol: 73mg

Sodium: 418mg

Carbs: 15g

Fiber: 2g

Sugar: 4g

Protein: 22g

Air Fryer Beef Kabobs

Serves- 4

Prep Time: 30 minutes

Cook Time: 10 minutes

Total Time: 40 minutes

Ingredients

1 lb. beef chuck ribs cut in 1-inch pieces

1/3 cup sour cream

2 tablespoon soy sauce

8 (6 –inch) skewers

1 bell peppers

½ onion

Directions

Preheat air fryer to 400^{0}F.

In a medium bowl, mix soy sauce and sour cream.

Add the beef chunks into the bowl; then marinate for 30 minutes at least or overnight.

Slice the bell pepper and onion into 1-inch pieces.

 Soak wooden skewers in water for about 10 minutes

Thread beef, onions, and bell peppers onto skewers.

Add some freshly ground black pepper.

Bake on preheated air fryer for 10 minutes, flipping halfway.

Serve.

Per Serving

Calories: 250

Carbs: 4g

Protein: 23g

Fat: 15g

Saturated Fat: 6g

Cholesterol: 84mg

Sodium: 609mg

Potassium: 519mg

Sugar: 2g

Garlic Roast Beef

Serves- 10

Prep Time: 5 minutes

Cook Time: 1 hour 15 minutes

Total Time: 2 hours 20 minutes

Ingredients

2-3 lb. roast or eye round, all fat trimmed off

Fresh cracked pepper, to taste

2 teaspoons dried chopped rosemary

3-4 cloves garlic, cut into thin slivers

Olive oil spray

Kosher salt, to taste

Directions

Take out the roast from the refrigerator 1 hour before cooking to be at room temperature.

Trim all the fat off the meat.

Piece the meat about ½ -inch deep with a sharp knife.

Insert the garlic slivers in each of the holes, push them inside very well.

Spray with olive oil lightly.

Season liberally with rosemary, pepper, and salt.

Arrange the meat into the air fryer basket, without touching each other.

Preheat air fryer at 350^0F for 10 to 20 minutes.

Insert the thermometer into the center of the meat to check the internal temperature at 165^0F.

Allow resting so that the juices are well distributed.

Slice thin and serve.

Per Serving

Calories: 142.5

Carbs: 0.5g

Protein: 24g

Fat: 4g

Cholesterol: 44mg

Sodium: 292.5mg

Fiber: 0.5g

Air Fried Beef Schnitzel

Serves- 1

Prep Time: 10minutes

Cook Time: 12min

Total Time: 22 minutes

Ingredients

2 tablespoon olive oil

50g breadcrumbs

1 egg, whisked

1 thin beef schnitzel

1 lemon, to serve

Directions

Preheat the air fryer to 355^{0}F.

Combine the olive oil and the breadcrumbs.

Continue to stir until the mixture is loose and crumble.

Dip the schnitzel into the egg then shake of any attachments.

Dip the schnitzel into the crumb mix ensuring that it is uniformly and completely coated.

Spread gently in the air fryer.

Cook for 12 minutes.

Serve and enjoy immediately with lemon.

Per Serving

Air Fryer Beef Casserole

Serves- 4

Prep Time: 29 minutes

Cook Time: 10 minutes

Total Time: 39 minutes

Ingredients

500 g beef tenderloin steak, cubed

1 tablespoon cornflour, divided

½ teaspoon each salt and pepper (approx.)

1 tablespoon olive oil

500 g new baby potatoes, quartered or cut into bite-sized pieces if large

500 ml seeded, chopped tomatoes

1 onion, thinly sliced

300 ml beef broth

1 tablespoon tomato paste

2 cloves garlic, minced

1 tablespoon minced fresh ginger root

750 ml baby arugula or spinach leaves

Directions

Add the beef cubes, pepper, half of the cornstarch, and salt together in a bowl; then toss.

Put the beef in the air fryer basket.

Drizzle evenly with half of the oil.

Cook at 350^{0}F for about 8 to 10 minutes or until browned.

Transfer the beef to a bowl and keep aside.

Add the tomatoes, potatoes, onion, broth, tomato paste, garlic, and the remaining oil to the air fryer basket.

Then bake for 40 minutes.

Toss the remaining cornflour with sufficient water to produce a creamy and smooth paste.

Stir into the stew and then bake for 5 minutes.

Add the ginger, the reserved beef, and any leftover juices.

Bake for 5 minutes or until beef is heated through and the potatoes are fork soft.

Stir in the arugula.

Fine-tune the seasoning with extra pepper if required.

Serve and enjoy!

Per Serving

CHAPTER 7

SEAFOOD

Fried Fish Nuggets

Serves- 4

Prep Time: 10 minutes

Cook Time: 10 minutes

Total Time: 20 minutes

Ingredients

1 lb. white fish (cod)

¼ cup mayonnaise

1½ cups pork rind panko

¾ teaspoon Cajun seasoning

2 tablespoons Dijon mustard

2 tablespoons water

Salt and pepper to taste

Directions

Spray the air fryer rack with nonstick cooking spray.

Pat the fish dry; then slice into sticks about 1-inch by 2-inches wide.

Toss the mustard, mayo, and water together in a small bowl.

In a different shallow, toss the pork rinds and Cajun seasoning together.

Season with pepper and salt to taste.

One by one dip into the mayo mixture to coat; tap to remove the excess.

Place on the air fryer rack.

Set an air fryer at 400^0F and bake for 5 minutes.

Use tongs to flip the fish sticks; then bake for an additional 5 minutes.

Serve immediately.

Per Serving

Calories: 263

Fat: 16g

Carbs: 1g

Fiber: 0.5g

Protein: 26.4g

Air Fryer Salmon With Maple Soy Glaze

Serves- 4

Prep Time: 5 minutes

Cook Time: 8 minutes

Total Time: 33 minutes

Ingredients

3 tablespoons pure maple syrup

3 tablespoons reduced-sodium soy sauce or gluten-free soy sauce

1 tablespoon sriracha hot sauce

1 clove garlic, smashed

4 wild salmon fillets, skinless (6 oz. each)

Directions

In a small bowl, combine the soy sauce, garlic, sriracha, and maple syrup.

Pour into a gallon-sized resealable bag or a Ziploc bag; then add the salmon.

Marinate for about 20 to 30 minutes, turning over intermittently.

Preheat air fryer to 400^0F.

Lightly spray the air fryer basket with nonstick spray.

Take the fish out of the marinade.

Pat dry with paper towels.

Reserve the marinade.

Put the fish in the air fryer in batches, cook for 7 to 8 minutes or longer based on the salmon thickness.

In the meantime, pour the marinade in a small saucepan.

Bring to a simmer over medium-low heat; then bring it down until thickens into a glaze about 1 to 2 minutes.

Spoon over the salmon just before eating.

Serve.

Per Serving

Calories: 292

Carbs: 12g

Protein: 35g

Fat: 11g

Saturated Fat:1.5g

Cholesterol: 94mg

Sodium: 797mg

Fiber: 0.5g

Sugar: 10g

Cajun Shrimp

Serves- 2

Total Time: 8 minutes

Ingredients

½ pound tiger shrimp

¼ teaspoon cayenne pepper

½ teaspoon old bay seasoning

¼ teaspoon smoked paprika

1 pinch of salt

1 tablespoon olive oil

Directions

Preheat the air fryer to 390°F.

Combine all of the ingredients in a mixing bowl.

Ensure that the shrimp is well coated with the oil and the spices.

Put the shrimp into the air fryer basket.

Bake for 5 minutes.

Serve and enjoy over cooked rice!

Per Serving

Air fried Salmon Patties

Serves- 6-8

Total Time:

Ingredients

3 large russet potatoes

1 salmon portion

Dashes of black pepper

Salt to taste

1 egg

Breadcrumbs (to coat)

Olive oil spray

A handful of frozen vegetables -parboiled and drained

Parsley, chopped

2 sprinkles of dill

Directions

Peel and cut the potatoes into bite-sized pieces.

Bring water to a boil in a pot.

Cook the potatoes in the water for nearly 10 minutes or until soft.

Drain off the water; return the potatoes to the pot on low heat.

Allow the water to evaporate, about 2 to 3 minutes, taking precautionary measures so that the potatoes do not burn.

Crush with a whisk; then add to a large bowl.

Chill until no more hot.

Meanwhile, prepare the breadcrumbs by blending it until fine; then keep aside.

Preheat the air fryer to 350^{0}F.

Grill the salmon for 5 minutes.

Use a fork to flake the salmon and then keep aside.

Take the mashed potatoes from the refrigerator; add parboiled veggies, chopped parsley, dill, black pepper, flaked salmon, and salt.

Adjust the seasonings to your taste.

Add the egg and mix everything.

Shape into 6 to 8 patties or smaller balls.

Coat with the breadcrumbs, then spray some oil as this will make the breadcrumbs to come out in pleasant colors.

Then air fry at 350^{0}F for 10 to 12 minutes or until golden.

Serve and enjoy with mayo and lemon as a salad on the side.

Per Serving

Coconut Shrimp with Spicy Marmalade Sauce

Serves-2

Prep Time: 10 minutes

Cook Time: 20 minutes

Total Time: 30 minutes

Ingredients

8 large shrimp shelled and deveined

8 ounces of coconut milk

½ cup shredded sweetened coconut

½ cup panko bread

½ teaspoon cayenne pepper

¼ teaspoon kosher salt

¼ teaspoon fresh ground pepper

½ cup orange marmalade

1 tablespoon honey

1 teaspoon mustard

¼ teaspoon hot sauce

Directions

Rinse the shrimp and keep aside.

Whisk the coconut milk in a small bowl.

Add the pepper and salt to season.

Keep aside.

In another small bowl, toss the panko, shredded coconut, pepper, salt, and cayenne pepper together.

One by one, dip the shrimp in the coconut milk, followed by panko.

Then set in the air fryer basket.

Repeat the procedure until all of the shrimp are coated.

Cook the shrimp in the air fryer for 20 minutes at 350^{0}F or until the shrimp are done.

In the meantime, as the shrimp are cooking, whisk the mustard, hot sauce, marmalade, and honey together in a bowl.

Serve the shrimp with the sauce immediately.

Per Serving

Calories: 623

Fat: 31g

Saturated Fat: 25g

Cholesterol: 82mg

Sodium: 864mg

Potassium: 348mg

Carbs: 76g

Fiber: 1g

Sugar: 57g

Protein: 15g

Air Fried Lemony White Fish and Garlic

Serves- 2

Prep Time: 5 minutes

Cook Time: 10 minutes

Total Time: 25 minutes

Ingredients

12 ounces tilapia filets, or other white fish

½ teaspoon onion powder, optional

Kosher salt, to taste

Fresh cracked black pepper, to taste

Fresh chopped parsley

Lemon wedges

½ teaspoon garlic powder

½ teaspoon lemon pepper seasoning

Directions

Pre-heat air fryer to 360°F for 5 minutes.

Wash and pat dry the fish fillets.

Coat with olive oil spray.

Season with lemon pepper, garlic powder, salt, pepper, and/or onion powder.

Repeat for both sides.

Spread punched air fryer baking paper in the base of the air fryer.

Spray the paper lightly.

On the other hand, if not using a liner, then spray sufficient olive oil spray at the base of the air fryer basket so that the fish will not be gummy.

Place the fish on top of the paper.

Add some lemon wedges besides the fish.

Set the air fryer to 360°F 6 to 12 minutes, or until fish can be flaked with a fork.

Take note that the thicker fillets will require a long time to bake.

Shower with chopped parsley.

Serve warm along with the toasted lemon wedges.

Per Serving

Air Fried Catfish

Serves- 4

Prep Time: 5 minutes

Cook Time: 1 hour

Total Time: 1 hour 5 minutes

Ingredients

4 catfish fillets

¼ cup seasoned fish fry

1 tablespoon olive oil

1 tablespoon chopped parsley (optional)

Directions

Pat the catfish dry.

Dust the seasoned fish fry onto both sides of each fillet.

Make sure the whole fillet is coated with the seasoning.

Drizzle the olive oil on the top of each fillet.

Put the fish fillet in the air fryer basket.

Don't overcrowd them.

Bake in batches if necessary.

Adjust the air fryer temperature to 350^0F at 10 minutes.

Close the air fryer and cook for 10 minutes.

Open the air fryer; then turn over the fish.

Bake for extra 10 minutes.

Then open and flip the fish again.

Cook for about 2 to 3 minutes more or until the desired doneness.

Top with parsley if preferred.

Serve.

Per Serving

Calories: 146

Fat: 3g

Saturated Fat: 1g

Cholesterol: 33mg

Sodium: 1741mg

Potassium: 400mg

Carbs: 18g

Fiber: 1g

Sugar: 11g

Protein: 11g

CHAPTER 8

SWEETS AND DESSERTS

Keto Chocolate Banana Brownie

Serves- 16

Prep Time: 5 minutes

Cook Time: 25 minutes

Total Time: 30 minutes

Ingredients

1 cup almond flour

3 Eggs

1/3 cup sugar-free chocolate chips

1 cup unsweetened peanut butter

½ cup of cocoa powder

¾ cup brown swerve sweetener

Directions

Add the eggs, pea butter, and brown swerve sweetener to a bowl; then whisk together.

Add in the cocoa powder, almond flour. Blend into a smooth batter.

Fold in chocolate chips into the batter.

Pour the batter into an oven-safe glass baking dish.

Put the oven-safe glass baking dish in the air fryer.

Cook for 25 minutes at 300^0F.

Serve.

Per Serving

Calories: 74

Protein: 3g

Fat: 6g

Carbs: 3g

Fiber:1g

Air Fried Keto Raspberry

Serve: 6

Prep Time: 10 minutes

Cook Time: 22 minutes

Total Time: 32 minutes

Ingredients

½ teaspoon orange zest

1/8 teaspoon salt

2½ tablespoons 40ml vegetable oil

1/3 cup sugar

1/3 cup milk

1 egg

1 cup plain flour

1 teaspoon baking powder

½ teaspoon vanilla essence

½ cup raspberries

½ tablespoon raw vanilla sugar

Directions

Place a paper muffin liner inside each cup of a muffin tray.

Mix the baking powder, flour, and salt in a large bowl.

Toss oil, vanilla, egg, sugar, and milk together in a different bowl until well mixed.

Add the wet ingredients into the dry ingredients; mix until just blended; then gently fold in the raspberry so that they don't break.

Share the muffin into muffin cups, top with vanilla sugar.

Set the air fryer to 350^0F at 12 to 15 minutes; then arrange the muffin cups into the air fryer basket in a single layer.

Bake for about 12 to 15 minutes or until a pin inserted into a muffin comes out clean.

Let the muffins cool a little bit in the baking tin before moving them to a rack to fully.

Serve.

Per Serving

Calories: 196

Carbs: 29g

Protein: 3g

Fat: 7g

Saturated Fat: 5g

Cholesterol: 28mg

Sodium: 66mg

Potassium: 138mg

Sugar: 12g

Keto Macaroon Fat Bomb

Serves- 30

Prep Time: 10 minutes

Cook Time: 20 minutes

Total Time: 45 minutes

Ingredients

2½ cups unsweetened desiccated coconut

2 large eggs

1 teaspoon vanilla essence

1½ cups coconut milk full fat

½ cup erythritol

⅓ cup coconut flour

Directions

Make a large cookie sheet by lining with parchment paper.

Combine all of the ingredients in a large bowl.

Blend very well into a thick batter.

Use a small-sized scoop to spoon the mixture onto the prepared cookie sheet.

Preheat air fryer to 350^0F.

Then place the prepared cookie sheet into the air fryer basket.

Bake for 15 to 20 minutes, until lightly browned.

Allow cooling

Leave to cool on the tray.

Enjoy the cooled cookies or store in an airtight container for later.

Per Serving

Calories: 80

Carbs: 3g

Protein: 1g

Fat: 8g

Saturated Fat: 6g

Cholesterol: 14mg

Sodium: 12mg

Potassium: 69mg

Fiber: 2g

Keto Lime Coconut Bars

Serves: 16

Total Time:

Ingredients

1 cup almond flour

3 tablespoons coconut flour

¼ cup swerve sweetener

Pinch salt

¼ cup coconut oil (melted)

Filling:

1 (15- oz.) can full-fat coconut milk

2/3 cup powdered swerve sweetener

½ teaspoon xanthan gum

½ cup lime juice

Lime zest (handful)

2 large eggs

Topping:

1/3 cup unsweetened flaked coconut (lightly toasted)

2 tablespoons powdered swerve sweetener

Directions

For the crust, preheat air fryer to 325^0F.

Combine the coconut flour, almond flour, salt, and sweetener.

Stir to blend very well.

Drizzle with melted coconut oil; then mix until well combined.

Press firmly and uniformly into the air fryer basket; arrange in a single layer.

Bake for about 8 to 10 minutes, until almost golden brown.

Remove and allow to cool whilst preparing the filling.

To make the filling, blend coconut milk and powdered sweetener in a saucepan over medium heat.

Bring to a boil; stir so that the sweetener can dissolve.

Shower the surface with xanthan gum; then toss very well to mix.

Allow cooling for at least 15 minutes.

Stir in the lime zest, lime juice, and the eggs.

Pour on top of the cooled crust in the air fryer.

Bake for 30 to 35 minutes or until the filling is just set though the center is still wiggled a little when shaken.

Chill until solid, about 2 hours.

Sprinkle with flaked coconut and powdered sweetener.

Enjoy!

Per Serving

Calories: 160

Total Fat: 13.8g

Saturated Fat: 5.9g

Cholesterol: 88mg

Sodium: 107mg

Potassium: 80mg

Carbs: 17.8g

Fiber: 2.1g

Sugar: 1g

Protein: 5.4g

Air fried Coconut Shrimp

Serves-

Prep Time: 10 minutes

Total Time: 20 minutes

Ingredients

½ cup all-purpose flour

1½ teaspoons black pepper

2 large eggs

2/3 cup unsweetened flaked coconut

1/3 cup panko (Japanese-style breadcrumbs)

12 ounces medium peeled, deveined raw shrimp, tail-on

Cooking spray

½ teaspoon kosher salt

1 serrano chili, thinly sliced

2 teaspoons chopped fresh cilantro (optional)

¼ cup honey

¼ cup lime juice

Directions

Blend the flour and the pepper in a shallow bowl.

In another shallow bowl, lightly beat eggs.

Stir panko and coconut together in a different shallow bowl.

Then dredge the shrimp into the flour mixture by holding each shrimp at the tail.

Be careful not to coat the tail and also shake off the excess.

Dip in egg, let any excess drip off.

Dredge in coconut mixture, pressing so that the coconut mixture can stick.

Coat shrimp well with cooking spray.

Put half of the shrimp in the air fryer basket.

Cook at 400°F for about 6 to 8 minutes, turning the shrimp over halfway through the cooking.

Season with ¼ teaspoon of the salt.

Repeat with the rest of the shrimp and salt.

Whilst the shrimp is cooking, toss lime juice, serrano chili, and honey together in a small bowl.

Sprinkle shrimp with cilantro, if preferred.

Serve with sauce.

Per Serving

Calories: 250

Fat: 9g

Saturated fat: 7g

Protein: 15g

Carbs: 30g

 Fiber: 2g

 Sugars: 18

Sodium: 527mg

Keto Thumbprint Cookies

Serve- 10

Prep Time: 15 minutes

Cook Time: 10 minutes

Total Time: 1 hour

Ingredients

1 cup almond flour

2 ounces cream cheese, softened

3 tablespoons low-calorie natural sweetener -swerve

1 egg

1 teaspoon baking powder

3 ½ tablespoons reduced-sugar raspberry preserves

Directions

Combine the almond flour, cream cheese, egg, baking powder, and sweetener in a bowl; then whisk so that a wet dough is formed.

Put the bowl in a freezer until the dough is cool enough that you can roll it into balls, about 20 minutes.

Preheat an air fryer to 400^{0}F in line with the manufacturer's instructions.

Line the basket with parchment paper.

Shape the dough into 10 balls.

Place them into the prepared basket.

Make a thumbprint in the center of each cookie.

Put 1 teaspoon of preserves into each indention.

Cook in the preheated air fryer until the edges are golden brown, about 7 minutes.

Cool cookies absolutely before moving from parchment paper, about 15 minutes, or else they will become a flaky mess

Serve.

Per Serving

Calories: 112

Total Fat: 8.6g

Saturated Fat: 1.9g

Cholesterol: 25mg

Sodium: 73mg

Potassium: 18mg

Carbs: 9.1g

Fiber: 1.4g

Sugar: 3g

Protein: 3.7g

Air Fried Simple Cookie

Serves- 2

Prep Time: 5 minutes

Cook Time: 7 minutes

Total Time: 12 minutes

Ingredients

2 teaspoon coconut flour

¼ teaspoon pink salt

1/8 teaspoon baking soda

1 large egg (room temperature)

¼ cup of chocolate chips

1 tablespoon butter, melted

1-2 tablespoon erythritol

10 drops liquid stevia

½ teaspoon vanilla extract

½ cup almond flour

Directions

In a medium bowl, combine all of the ingredients apart from the chocolate chips and whisk to blend; then let it alone for about 2 to 3 minutes.

Line the bottom of the air fryer with a piece of parchment paper.

Fold the chocolate chips into the dough.

Preheat the air fryer to 350°F for 2 minutes (without the parchment paper) and then turn off.

Set the dough onto the parchment paper and spread using a spatula to ¼ inch thickness or place another sheet of parchment paper on top and roll out.

Remove the air fryer basket; then put the parchment paper in the preheated air fryer.

Cook for 5 to 10 minutes.

Make sure you keep an eye on it as the air fryer cooking times vary greatly.

Remove parchment paper from the air fryer to a plate.

Serve immediately.

Per Serving

Calories: 273

Fat: 28g

Carbs: 15g

Fiber: 9g

Protein: 11g

Cherry Pie Bars

Serve- 2

Prep Time: 5 minutes

Cook Time: 17 minutes

Total Time: 22 minutes

Ingredients

3 cups cherries pitted and halved

2 tablespoons maple syrup

1 tablespoon non-dairy butter melted

½ teaspoon almond extract optional

4 tablespoons crispy granola

Directions

Preheat the air fryer to 350^0F.

Combine cherries, non-dairy butter, almond extract (if using), and maple syrup.

Then add to the air fryer safe baking dish.

Put the cherry crisp into the air fryer.

Cook for 15 minutes or until the cherries are cooked to your desire.

Stir the cherry mixture at least once during cooking.

Once it is cooked through, open the air fryer basket; then add granola on top of the cooked cherries.

Then cook for an additional 2 to 3 minutes.

Serve and enjoy warm with non-dairy ice cream on the side.

Per Serving

Calories: 316

Carbs: 62g

Protein: 4g

Fat: 7g

Saturated Fat: 1g

Sodium: 48mg

Potassium: 505mg

Fiber: 6g

Sugar: 43g

Air Fried Roasted Almonds

Serve- 4

Prep Time: 1 minute

Cook Time: 8 minutes

Total Time: 9 minutes

Ingredients

1 cup whole raw almonds with skins on

Directions

Preheat the air fryer to 350^0F.

Put the raw almonds into the air fryer basket, ensuring that they are in a single layer.

You can cook them in batches if there is a need.

Cook for 5 to 8 minutes, turning halfway through.

Check after 5 minutes and cook for an extra 2 to 3 minutes or until done to your preference.

Let the roasted almonds; then serve.

Per Serving

Calories: 206

 Carbs: 8g

 Protein: 8g

 Fat: 18g

 Saturated Fat: 1g

 Sodium: 1mg

Potassium: 252mg

 Fiber: 4g

 Sugar: 1g

 Nutella Smores

Serve- 4

Prep Time: 2 minutes

Cook Time: 5 minutes

Total Time: 7 minutes

Ingredients

4 graham crackers cut in half (or 8 biscuits of your liking)

4 jumbo marshmallows

A handful of Strawberries and Raspberries

4 teaspoons of Nutella

Directions

Preheat the air fryer to 350^0F.

Place 4 graham cracker halves or 4 biscuits in the air fryer basket.

Place 1 marshmallow on top of each graham cracker half.

Cook for 5 minutes, until marshmallow, is pleasant and golden.

Add the berries and the Nutella.

Top each with a graham cracker half (or biscuit).

Serve.

 Enjoy!

Per Serving

Calories: 172

Carbs: 35g

Protein: 1g

Fat: 2g

Saturated Fat: 1g

Sodium: 115mg

Potassium: 63mg

Sugar: 21g

Chocolate Cake

Serve- 10

Prep Time: 10 minutes

Cook Time: 55 minutes

Total Time: 1 hour 5 minutes

Directions

3 large eggs

1 cup almond flour

2/3 cup sugar

1/3 cup heavy cream

¼ cup coconut oil melted

¼ cup unsweetened cocoa powder

1 teaspoon baking powder

½ teaspoon orange zest

1/8 cup chopped walnuts

1/8 cup chopped pecans

Unsalted butter (at room temperature)

Directions

Butter a 7-inch round baking pan and line the bottom with parchment paper.

Put all of the ingredients into a large bowl.

Use a hand mixer on medium speed to beat until batter is fluffy and light.

This is essential so that the cake won't be too heavy.

Carefully fold the nuts into the batter to keep the air in.

Pour cake batter into the pan and cover firmly with aluminum foil.

Set in the air fryer basket and cook for 45 minutes at 325^0F.

Remove the foil.

Then cook for an extra 10 to 15 minutes, until a pin or knife inserted in the middle comes out clean.

Remove the pan out of the air fryer and place it on a cooling rack for 10 minutes.

Then remove the cake from the pan and allow it to cool for an additional 20 minutes.

Slice.

Serve

Per Serving

Calories: 232

 Carbs: 17g

 Protein: 4g

Fat: 17g

Saturated Fat: 7g

Cholesterol: 59mg

Sodium: 22mg

 Potassium: 119mg

 Fiber: 2g

 Sugar: 13g

Apple Chips

Serve- 2

Prep Time: 10 minutes

Cook Time: 20 minutes

Total Time: 30 minutes

Ingredients

1 apple

¼ teaspoon ground cinnamon

Pinch of salt

Directions

Preheat the air fryer to 350^{0}F.

Slice the apples thinly with the help of a sharp knife or a mandolin.

Put the apple slices in a bowl; then add cinnamon and salt.

Whisk to combine.

Add half of the spiced apple slices to the air fryer basket.

Make sure they are arranged in a single layer.

Cook for 8 to 10 minutes, turning and flattening them at least 2 times during the cooking.

Remove the cooked apple chips.

Then repeat with the remaining spiced apple slices.

Serve.

Per Serving

Calories: 48

Carbs: 12g

Potassium: 97mg

Fiber: 2g

Sugar: 9g

Roasted Spicy Peanuts

Serve- 4

Prep Time: 5 minutes

Cook Time: 10 minutes

Total Time: 15 minutes

Ingredients

2 cups of raw peanuts (shelled)

¼ cup of sugar

1 teaspoon smoked paprika

1 tablespoon melted butter

Directions

Add the raw peanuts to a large bowl.

Add the smoked paprika and the sugar; then whisk so that the peanuts are fully coated.

Add the melted butter.

Mix well so that the peanuts can be coated.

 Add a piece of parchment paper to the air fryer basket.

Then layer the peanuts on the air fryer basket.

Set the air fryer at 300^{0}F for 5 minutes.

Remove after it is cooked through or add extra 5 minutes if not satisfied in the first place.

Serve and enjoy!

Per Serving

Spicy Roasted Cashew Nuts

Serves- 3

Prep Time: 5 minutes

Cook Time: 10 minutes

Total Time: 15 minutes

Ingredients

1 teaspoon smoked paprika

1 teaspoon ground coriander

1 teaspoon ground cumin

3 cups of cashews (either half or whole)

1 teaspoon kosher salt

2 tablespoons olive oil

Directions

Put the cashews, the smoked paprika, ground cumin, salt, olive oil, and ground coriander in a small bowl.

Whisk together so that cashews are coated very well.

Spread the cashews on either the air fryer tray or air fryer basket.

Place the tray or basket into the air fryer.

Adjust the air fryer to 330^0F at 5 minutes.

Remove to a serving plate or bowl.

Serve.

Enjoy!

Doritos Chips

Serves- 3

Prep Time: 5 minutes

Cook Time: 7 minutes

Total Time: 12 minutes

Ingredients

1 teaspoon chili powder

1 teaspoon smoked paprika

1 teaspoon salt

6 corn tortillas

2 tablespoons melted butter

3 tablespoons grated parmesan cheese

Directions

Melt butter in a small ramekin.

Mix the chili powder, parmesan cheese, smoked paprika, and salt in a resealable bag.

Brush the butter over all the corn tortilla on both sides using a pastry brush.

Use a pizza cutter to cut the corn tortillas into triangles.

Then dip the triangle corn tortillas in the cheese mixture, ensuring that both sides are fully coated.

Spray the air fryer basket or tray with nonstick cooking spray.

The set the coated corn tortillas into an air fryer basket or tray.

Set the temperature for 300^{0}F, for 5 minutes.

(Then quickly spray of olive oil, on the corn tortillas).

Allow them to cool, they will harden as they cool.

Remove to plate.

Serve and enjoy!

Per Serving

Blueberry Scones

Serves- 8

Prep Time: 5 minutes

Cook Time: 12 minutes

Total Time: 17 minutes

Ingredients

½ stick cold unsalted butter

¼ cup heavy cream

1 egg

1 teaspoon pure vanilla extract

½ cup fresh blueberries

1 cup flour

¼ cup of sugar

1 teaspoon baking powder

1 teaspoon ground cinnamon

½ teaspoon salt

Directions

Mix the ground cinnamon, baking powder, sugar, flour, and salt in a large bowl.

Then stir in the butter, heavy cream, eggs, and vanilla extract; mix very well.

Fold in the blueberries; mix very well until they are well scattered.

Generously spray your scone pan (either one you are using) with olive oil.

Fill the pan with the batter.

See to it that it is sure to get the corners and then press well.

Place the pan or the scone silicone molds into the air fryer.

Put the temperature to 320^0F for 12 minutes.

Take note that the exact time depends on the air fryer model.

Ensure that they are completely cooked before you pop them out.

Remove to the plate.

Serve and enjoy!

Per Serving

CONCLUSION

Eating healthy is never an abrupt choice to make but a lasting lifestyle change that impacts one's state of mind. In this wise, individuals must endeavor to make informed decisions and stay true to their health goals. We quite realize that these days scores of temptation are around the corner to lure people off their commitments.

The air fryer will inspire you to enjoy cooking healthy and well-balanced meals for yourself, family, and friends all the time. Recent findings have revealed that air-fried foods have about 80 percent less fat as against deep-fried foods. Deep-fried foods are the major contributor to type 2 diabetes, overweight/obesity, increased risk of cardiovascular disease, high cholesterol, etc. Besides, fats and oils tend to become toxic under high heat thus causing inflammation of the body and increased premature aging. Similarly, these oils released carcinogens that are harmful to body cells.

However, studies have confirmed that healthy fats and oils are exceptionally beneficial most especially if you are on a keto diet. Ensure that you stay away from hydrogenated oils and genetically modified oils, for example, rice bran oil, cottonseed oil, soybean oil, and corn oil. Avoid margarine too because it contains trans-fats. Good fats and oils include avocado oil, olive oil, coconut oil, sesame oil, seeds, and nuts.

Air-fried foods are yummy and have a texture similar to common fried foods only that they taste differently.

Air fryer as a wonderful kitchen appliance will help fast track your weight loss goals.

Part 2

GARLIC PARMESAN CHICKEN WINGS

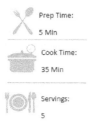

Prep Time:
5 Min

Cook Time:
35 Min

Servings:
5

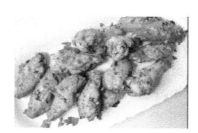

INGREDIENTS:

- 2 lemons, thinly sliced
- 1 large salmon fillet (about 3 lb.)
- Kosher salt
- Freshly ground black pepper
- 6 tbsp. butter, melted
- 2 tbsp. honey
- 3 cloves garlic, minced
- 1 tsp. chopped thyme leaves
- 1 tsp. dried oregano
- Chopped fresh parsley, for garnish

DIRECTIONS:

1. Take the chicken wing parts out of the refrigerator and pat them dry.

2. Mix sea salt, black pepper, bell pepper, garlic powder, onion powder and baking powder in a small bowl.
3. Sprinkle the spice mixture on the wings and throw it to cover.
4. Place the wings on a flat layer in the air fryer.
5. Use the chicken air fryer (400 degrees) and cook for 30 minutes. To make the wings crispy quickly, you have to turn them about halfway.
6. Mix all the ingredients for the garlic parmesan sauce by stirring them in a small bowl.
7. Put the wings in the garlic-parmesan mixture and serve immediately.

AIR FRYER KETO BUFFALO CHICKEN WINGS

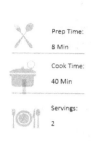

Prep Time:
8 Min

Cook Time:
40 Min

Servings:
2

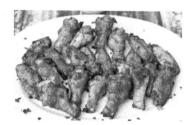

INGREDIENTS:

- 1 2/3 c. almond flour
- 2 tbsp. flaxseed meal
- 2 tbsp. coconut flour
- 2 tsp. baking soda
- 1/2 tsp. kosher salt
- 5 large eggs
- 1/4 c. extra-virgin olive oil
- 1 tbsp. agave syrup
- 1 tbsp. apple cider vinegar
  >

DIRECTIONS:

1. Take the chicken wing parts out of the refrigerator and pat them dry.
2. Mix sea salt, black pepper, paprika, garlic powder, onion powder and baking powder in a small bowl or baking dish

3. Sprinkle the spice mixture on the wings and throw it to cover
4. Place the wings on a flat layer in the air fryer
5. Use the chicken air fryer (400 degrees) and cook for 30 minutes. To make the wings crispy quickly, you have to turn them about halfway.
6. Mix all of the ingredients for the Buffalo Wing sauce by stirring them in a small bowl with a fork (keep mixing until the melted butter is well incorporated).
7. Put the wings in the buffalo sauce mixture and serve immediately.

KETO BUFFALO CAULIFLOWER BITES

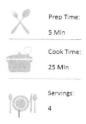

Prep Time:
5 Min

Cook Time:
25 Min

Servings:
4

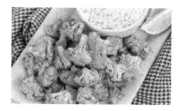

INGREDIENTS:

- 3 tbsp. extra-virgin olive oil, divided
- 3 swordfish steaks
- kosher salt
- Freshly ground black pepper
- 2 pt. multicolored cherry tomatoes, halved
- 1/4 c. red onion, finely chopped
- 3 tbsp. Thinly sliced basil
- Juice of 1/2 a lemon

DIRECTIONS:

For the air fryer

Cut the cauliflower into florets of equal size and place in a large bowl.

1. Cut each clove of garlic into 3 pieces and smash them with the side of your knife. Don't be afraid to smash the garlic. You want to expose as much of the garlic

surface as possible so that it cooks well. Add this to the cauliflower.
2. Pour over the oil and add salt. Mix well until the cauliflower is well covered with oil and salt.
3. Turn on the air fryer at 400 F for 20 minutes and add the cauliflower. Turn it in half once.

MAKE THE SAUCE

1. While the cauliflower is cooking, make the sauce. Whisk the hot sauce, butter and Worcestershire sauce in a small bowl.
2. Once the cauliflower is cooked, place it in a large bowl. Pour the hot sauce over the cauliflower and mix well.
3. Put the cauliflower back in the air fryer. Set it to 400F for 3-4 minutes so the sauce becomes a little firm.
4. Serve with blue cheese dressing.

SPICY DRY-RUBBED CHICKEN WINGS

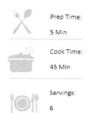

Prep Time:
5 Min

Cook Time:
45 Min

Servings:
6

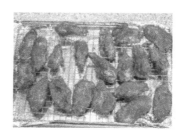

INGREDIENTS:

- 4 6-oz. skin-on salmon fillets
- Extra-virgin olive oil, for brushing
- kosher salt
- Freshly ground black pepper
- 2 lemons, sliced
- 2 tbsp. butter

DIRECTIONS:

Marinating the wings:

1. Take the chicken out of the fridge and let it approach room temperature (30 minutes). Preheat the oven to 400 degrees.
2. Place the chicken in a Ziploc sachet with 1/4 cup of the spicy dry massage. You can keep the rest in a mason jar.
3. Shake the bag so that the mixture covers the chicken evenly.

4. Store in the refrigerator for at least four hours, ideally overnight.

AIR FRYER STEAK BITES AND MUSHROOMS

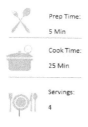

Prep Time:
5 Min

Cook Time:
25 Min

Servings:
4

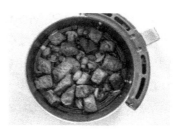

INGREDIENTS:

- 2 tbsp. extra-virgin olive oil
- 1 medium onion, chopped
- 1 bell pepper, chopped
- 3 cloves garlic, minced
- 1 tbsp. tomato paste
- 1 lb. Italian sausage
- 1 tbsp. chili powder
- 1 tsp. dried oregano
- 1/2 tsp. garlic powder
- 1/4 tsp. cayenne
- Kosher salt
- Freshly ground black pepper
- 4 large sweet potatoes, peeled and cubed into 1" pieces
- 3 c. low-sodium chicken broth
- 1 (14.5-oz.) can diced tomatoes
- Freshly chopped parsley, for serving

DIRECTIONS:

1. Preheat the empty air fryer to 390 ° F with a crisp plate or basket for 4 minutes.
2. Pat the meat dry. As the air fryer heats up, throw beef cubes with olive oil and Montreal spices.
3. Halve or halve mushrooms. Pour beef cubes and mushrooms into the preheated air fryer and gently shake to combine.
4. Set the air fryer temperature to 390 ° F and the timer for 8 minutes.
5. Stop after 3 minutes and shake the basket. Repeat this process every 2 minutes until the beef cubes have reached the desired degree of cooking. Lift a large piece out and test it with a meat thermometer or cut and look in the middle to see the progress. Note that the meat will continue to cook as soon as it is removed from the air fryer and resting. Meat is medium at 145 ° F and has a warm pink center.
6. Let the meat rest for a few minutes before serving and then enjoy

PECAN CRUSTED CHICKEN

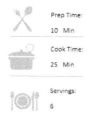

Prep Time:
10 Min

Cook Time:
25 Min

Servings:
6

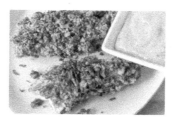

INGREDIENTS:

- 3 breakfast sausage patties
- 1 avocado, mashed
- kosher salt
- Freshly ground black pepper
- 3 large eggs
- chives, for garnish
- Hot sauce, if desired

DIRECTIONS:

1. Place the chicken tenders in a large bowl.
2. Add salt, pepper and smoked paprika and mix well until the chicken is covered with the spices.
3. Pour in honey and mustard and mix well.
4. Place the finely chopped pecans on a plate.
5. Roll the tender into the shredded pecans, one chicken tender at a time, until both sides are covered. Brush off excess material.

6. Place the offers in the air fryer basket and continue until all offers have been coated and are in the air fryer basket.
7. Set the air fryer to 350F for 12 minutes until the chicken is cooked through and the pecans are golden brown before serving.

CHICKEN TIKKA KEBAB

Prep Time:
10 Min

Cook Time:
30Min

Serving:
6

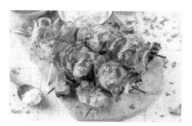

INGREDIENTS:

- 1 bell pepper, sliced into 1/4" rings
- 6 eggs
- kosher salt
- Freshly ground black peppers
- 2 tbsp. Chopped chives
- 2 tbsp. chopped parsley

DIRECTIONS:

1. Mix all the ingredients for the marinade in a bowl and mix well. Add chicken and spread the marinade on each side. Let it rest in the fridge for between 30 minutes and 8 hours.
2. Add oil, onions, green and red peppers to the marinade for cooking. Mix well.
3. Thread the marinated chicken, peppers and onions into the skewers in between.

   Air Fryer method:

1. Lightly grease the air fryer basket.
2. Arrange the chicken sticks in the Air fryer. Cook them at 180 degrees for 10 minutes.
3. Turn the chicken sticks and cook for another 7 minutes, then serve.

AIR FRYER PIZZA

Prep Time:
10 Min

Cook Time:
25 Min

Servings:
6

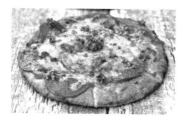

INGREDIENTS:

- 2 5-oz. cans tuna, drained
- 1/4 c. mayonnaise
- 1 tbsp. Dijon mustard
- 2 stalks celery, finely chopped
- Juice of 1/2 a lemon
- 1 tbsp. chopped dill, plus more for garnish
- kosher salt
- Freshly ground black pepper
- 6 dill pickles
- Paprika, for garnish

DIRECTIONS:

1. Preparation: Preheat the air fryer to 190 ° C. Spray the air fryer basket well with oil. Pat mozzarella dry with paper towels (to prevent a wet pizza).
2. Assemble: Roll out the pizza dough to the size of your air fryer basket. Transfer it gently into the air fryer, then lightly brush it with a teaspoon of olive oil. Pour a

173

light layer of tomato sauce on top and sprinkle with buffalo mozzarella.
3. Bake: for about 7 minutes until the crust is crisp and the cheese has melted. Optionally, topping with basil, grated parmesan and pepper flakes shortly before serving.

AIR FRYER BRUSSELS SPROUTS

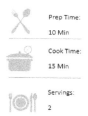

Prep Time:
10 Min

Cook Time:
15 Min

Servings:
2

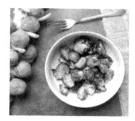

INGREDIENTS:

- 1/4 c. balsamic vinegar
- 3 tbsp. extra-virgin olive oil
- 2 tbsp. brown sugar
- 3 cloves garlic, minced
- 1 tsp. dried thyme
- 1 tsp. dried rosemary
- 4 chicken breasts
- Kosher salt
- Freshly ground black pepper
- Freshly chopped parsley, for garnish

DIRECTIONS:

1. Preparation: remove the hard ends of the Brussels sprouts and remove any damaged outer leaves. Rinse under cold water and pat dry. If your sprouts are large, cut them in half. Add oil, salt and pepper.
2. Cooking: Arrange Brussels sprouts in a single layer in your air fryer and work in batches if not all fit. Cook for 8 to 12 minutes at 190 ° C and shake the pan halfway

through the cooking process to brown it evenly. They are done when they are lightly browned and crispy at the edges.
3. Serving: Serve sprouts warm, optionally with balsamic reduction and parmesan

CRISPY AIR FRIED TOFU

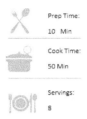

Prep Time:
10 Min

Cook Time:
50 Min

Servings:
8

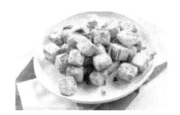

INGREDIENTS:

- 2 c. almond flour
- 1/2 tsp. baking soda
- 1/4 tsp. kosher salt
- 1/4 c. butter, room temperature
- 1/4 c. almond butter
- 3 tbsp. honey
- 1 large egg
- 1 tsp. pure vanilla extract
- 1 c. semisweet chocolate chips
- Flaky sea salt

DIRECTIONS:

1. Squeeze: Squeeze the tofu for at least 15 minutes by placing either a heavy pan or a pan on top and letting the moisture drain. When you're done, cut the tofu into bite-sized blocks and put it in a bowl.
2. Taste: Mix all remaining ingredients in a small bowl. Drizzle over the tofu and toss to cover. Let the tofu marinate for another 15 minutes.

3. Air fryer: Preheat your air fryer to 190 ° C. Add tofu blocks to your air fryer basket in a single layer. Let cook for 10 to 15 minutes and shake the pan occasionally to promote even cooking.

BUTTERMILK FRIED MUSHROOMS

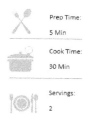

Prep Time:
5 Min

Cook Time:
30 Min

Servings:
2

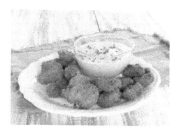

INGREDIENTS:

- 1 lb. shrimp
- 2 tbsp. olive oil
- 1 tsp. kosher salt
- 1 tsp. cayenne
- 1 tsp. paprika
- 1 tsp. garlic powder
- 1 tsp. onion powder
- 1 tsp. oregano
- 2 lemons, sliced thinly crosswise

DIRECTIONS:

1. Marinate: Preheat the air fryer to 190 ° C. Clean the mushrooms and place in a large bowl with buttermilk. Let marinate for 15 minutes.
2. Breading: Mix the flour and spices in a large bowl. Put the mushrooms out of the buttermilk (keep the buttermilk). Dip each mushroom in the flour mixture,

shake off excess flour, dip again in the buttermilk and then again in the flour (short: wet> dry> wet> dry).

3. Cooking: Grease the bottom of your air pan well and place the mushrooms in a layer, leaving space between the mushrooms. Let it cook for 5 minutes, then roughly coat all sides with a little oil to promote browning. Cook for another 5 to 10 minutes until golden brown and crispy.

AIR FRYER POTATOES

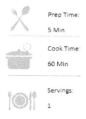

Prep Time:
5 Min

Cook Time:
60 Min

Servings:
1

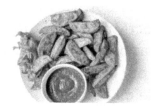

INGREDIENTS:

- 1 head green cabbage, rinsed and sliced very thinly;
- 1 large carrot, shredded;
- 2 cups fresh pineapple, peeled, cored and chopped;
- 1 cup mandarin oranges, chopped;
- 1 cup red grapes, chopped;
- 1/4 cup homemade mayonnaise;
- Fruity Coleslaw preparation

DIRECTIONS:

Air Fryer baked potatoes

1. Preparation: Preheat the air fryer to 200 ° C. Rub potatoes with a little vegetable oil and sprinkle with salt.
2. Cooking: Put the potatoes in one layer in the air fryer. Let it cook for 30 to 45 minutes or until the fork is soft. Turn once during baking to cook evenly.

Air fryer French fries

1. 1 Soak: Cut potatoes into matches with a knife or a mandolin cutter. Soak sliced potatoes in a bowl of cold water for 1 hour. This will remove starch to give them the perfectly crispy texture!
2. 2 Preparation: Preheat the air fryer to 200 ° C. Drain and dab dry potatoes. Place in a bowl and drizzle with vegetable oil and a pinch of salt.
3. 3 Cooking: add fries to your air fryer and spread them in one layer as possible. Let cook for 15 to 20 minutes, shaking the basket a few times to cook evenly.

CRISPY BAKED AVOCADO TACOS

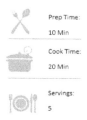

Prep Time:
10 Min

Cook Time:
20 Min

Servings:
5

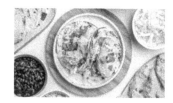

INGREDIENTS:

- 6 slices of ham (we used Applegate brand)
- 4 eggs
- 1/4 cup full-fat coconut milk
- 1/4 cup orange bell peppers, chopped
- 1/4 cup red bell peppers, chopped
- 1/4 cup yellow onions, chopped
- Salt & pepper, to taste
- Olive oil or coconut oil to sauté veggies

DIRECTIONS:

1. Salsa: Combine all the salsa ingredients and put them in the fridge.
2. Prepare avocado: Halve the length of the avocado and remove the pit. Lay the avocado skin face down and cut each half into 4 equal pieces. Then gently peel off the skin.
3. Preparation station: Preheat the oven to 230 ° C or the air fryer to 190 ° C. Arrange your work area so that you have a bowl of flour, a bowl of whisk, a bowl of Panko

with S&P, and a baking sheet lined with parchment at the end.

4. Coat: Dip each avocado slice first in the flour, then in the egg and then in the panko. Place on the prepared baking sheet and bake for 10 minutes or fry in the air. Lightly brown after half of the cooking process.

5. Sauce: While cooking avocados, combine all the sauce ingredients.

6. Serve: Put salsa on a tortilla, top with 2 pieces of avocado and drizzle with sauce. Serve immediately and enjoy!

AIR FRYER KALE CHIPS

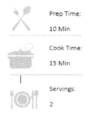

Prep Time:
10 Min

Cook Time:
15 Min

Servings:
2

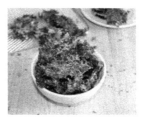

INGREDIENTS:

- 2 cups seven-grain hot cereal
- 1 medium apple, peeled and chopped
- 1/4 cup dried apricots, chopped
- 1/4 cup dried cranberries
- 1/4 cup chopped dates
- 1/4 cup raisins
- 1 teaspoon ground cinnamon
- 1/2 teaspoon salt
- 5 cups water
- 1 cup unsweetened apple juice
- 1/4 cup maple syrup
- Chopped walnuts

DIRECTIONS:

1. Preparation: Wash and dry kale. Cut the leaves off the spine and roughly tear them into bite-sized pieces. Massage oil into the leaves, making sure that each piece of kale has a thin layer of oil. Sprinkle with salt and throw to cover.

2. Transfer: Put kale in a single layer in your air fryer basket and loosen the leaves as much as possible without overlapping too much (you may need to cook in batches).
3. Cooking: Fry in the air for 4 to 5 minutes at 190 ° C and shake the pan once so that it can cook evenly. Keep an eye on them after 3 minutes. They're done when they're crispy!

AIR FRYER SWEET POTATO FRIES

Prep Time:
10 Min

Cook Time:
60 Min

Servings:
4

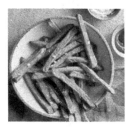

INGREDIENTS:

- 1 sweet potato
- 1 tsp olive oil 5 ml
- Pinch of salt

DIRECTIONS:

1. Cutting: To cut traditional fries, cut your sweet potato lengthways into thin boards and cut each board into strips. To cut sweet potato wedges, cut your sweet potato lengthways in half. Cut the length again in half and then each of these halves again in half. (Each potato should make 8 wedges, although you can cut them smaller if your sweet potato is large).
2. Soak: Soak the fries in cold water for 30 to 60 minutes before frying them in the air.
3. Drying: Drain the sweet potato wedges and pat dry. Place in a bowl and drizzle with vegetable oil (approx. 1 teaspoon per potato) and a pinch of salt.

4. Air roast: add fries to your air fryer and spread them in one layer as possible. Cook for 15 to 20 minutes at 200 ° C and shake every few minutes to cook evenly.

Prep Time:
10 Min

Cook Time:
25 Min

Servings:
4

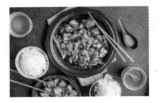

BAKED GENERAL TSO'S CAULIFLOWER

INGREDIENTS:

- Cauliflower
- ½ head cauliflower
- ½ cup flour 60g
- 2 large eggs whisked
- cup panko breadcrumbs 50 g
- ¼ tsp each salt and pepper
- General Tso's Sauce
- Tbsp sesame oil 15 ml
- cloves garlic minced
- Tbsp fresh grated ginger
- ½ cup vegetable broth 120 ml
- ¼ cup soy sauce 60 ml
- ¼ cup rice vinegar 60 ml
- ¼ cup brown sugar 50 g

- Tbsp tomato paste 30 g
- Tbsp cornstarch dissolved in 2 Tbsp (30 ml) cold water 15 g

DIRECTIONS:

1. Preparation: Preheat the oven to 204 ° C *. Arrange the work area and put flour, egg and panko in separate bowls. Mix salt and pepper in panko. Cut cauliflower into bite-sized florets.
2. Dredging: Brush the florets in batches with flour, then with egg and then with breadcrumbs. Place on a baking sheet lined with parchment paper. Bake for 15 to 20 minutes or until crispy.
3. Sauce: Place a small saucepan over medium heat and add the sesame oil, garlic and ginger. Let it cook for 2 minutes until it smells, then add the remaining ingredients to the sauce except the cornstarch mixture. Whisk to mix and bring to a boil. Pour in the cornstarch mixture slowly while stirring. It should thicken fairly quickly; If not, keep simmering until thick.
4. Assemble: Drizzle the sauce over the baked cauliflower and stir gently to spread it evenly. Serve cauliflower over warm rice or quinoa.

CPSIA information can be obtained
at www.ICGtesting.com
Printed in the USA
BVHW030925120922
646800BV00016B/437